PCOS AND HAIR HARMONY

A Simple Guide to Understanding the Connection & Managing It Effectively

KHADIJA MUSTAFA

First Edition 2024

Published by Khadija Mustafa

TABLE OF CONTENTS

CHAPTER 3: NAVIGATING HORMONAL IMBALANCES

CHAPTER 4: TREATMENT FOR HAIR RELATED ISSUES IN PCOS

- Plucking
- Waxing
- Bleaching
- Depilatory Creams
- Laser Hair Removal
- IPL (Intense Pulsed Light) Therapy
- Electrolysis

CHAPTER 5: MAINTENANCE OF HAIR & PCOS HOLLISTICAL

1. Dietary Changes
2. Food that can worsen PCOS symptoms
3. Glycemic Index
- Low-GI Diet
- High-GI Diet
4. Nutritional Supplements for PCOS and Hair
5. Physical Activity
6. Importance of Exercise
7. Types of Exercise
- Aerobic Exercise
- Resistance Training
- Meditation
- Breathing Exercise
- Yoga and Pilates
8. Exercise Routine Recommendations
9. Incorporating Enjoyable Activities to Maintain Consistency

CHAPTER 6: PCOS PSYCHOLOGICAL WELL-BEING AND HAIR HEALTH

1. Importance of Addressing Psychological Well-Being in Managing PCOS-Related Hair Concerns
2. Emotional Challenges Associated with PCOS Diagnosis
- Diagnosis Shock and Uncertainty
- Body Image Issues

- Fertility Concerns
- Social Stigma and Isolation

3. Impact of Hormonal Imbalances on Mood, Self-Esteem, And Body Image In PCOS

4. Psychological Effects of Hair Loss in PCOS

5. Psychological Effects of Hirsutism in PCOS

6. Coping Mechanisms for Managing Hair-Related Psychological Issues in PCOS

7. Strategies for Coping with Emotional Challenges and Achieving Hair Harmony

8. Role of Healthcare Providers in Addressing Psychological Concerns and Providing Emotional Support

CHAPTER 7: DIY RECIPES TO MANAGE PCOS AND HAIR HEALTH

1. Recipes for Hormonal Balance in PCOS

2. Recipes for Hair Loss in PCOS

3. Recipes for Hirsutism in PCOS

CHAPTER 1:

UNDERSTANDING PCOS

1. What are Polycystic Ovaries?
2. What happens in the ovaries?
3. Difference between Polycystic Ovary and Polycystic Ovarian Syndrome
4. Symptoms of PCOS
   - Emotions
   - Insulin Resistance
   - Fertility Problem
   - Period Disruption
   - Weight Gain
   - Different Hair Patterns
   - Fatigue
   - Pain
   - Skin Changes
   - Acne and Oily Skin
   - Depression
5. PCOS through life's changes

Forget skimming the entire book – this chapter is your PCOS one-stop-shop! Whether you're newly diagnosed, suspecting PCOS, or supporting a loved one, this overview unveils everything you need to know. Dive deep into the condition itself, its diverse symptoms, and most importantly, empowering treatment options you can implement right away.

But this isn't just another medical guide. We go beyond the basics to explore the hair connection — a vital aspect of PCOS often overlooked. Discover how this condition can impact your hair growth, texture, and thickness, and unlock personalized strategies to combat these concerns. Take charge of your well-being and embrace healthier, happier hair alongside effective PCOS management. This chapter equips you with the knowledge and tools to thrive, not just survive.

UNDERSTANDING PCOS:

PCOS, short for Polycystic Ovary Syndrome, isn't just a medical term; it's a reality for millions of women worldwide. Affecting 5-10% of women in their childbearing years, it's the most common hormonal disorder during this time. But it's crucial to understand that not everyone with polycystic ovaries (PCOs) has PCOS. While 20% of women have PCOs without displaying symptoms, PCOS is diagnosed only when specific symptoms are present.

While the exact cause of PCOS remains a mystery, we do know it's influenced by a combination of genetics and environmental factors. And the good news? You're not alone in navigating this journey. With the right understanding and proactive approach, you can manage PCOS effectively and reclaim your well-being.

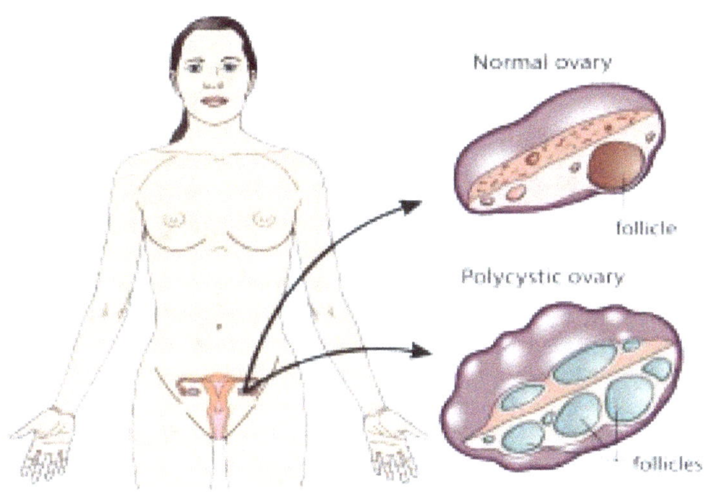

WHAT ARE POLYCYSTIC OVARIES?

Polycystic ovaries are slightly larger than normal ovaries and have twice the number of follicles (fluid-filled spaces within the ovary that release the eggs when you ovulate).

WHAT HAPPENS IN THE OVARIES?

PCOS, or Polycystic Ovary Syndrome, is a health condition that primarily affects the reproductive system in individuals with ovaries. Therefore, it occurs in the ovaries. In PCOS, the ovaries may contain small, undeveloped follicles, forming cysts. These cysts can disrupt the normal functioning of the ovaries and contribute to hormonal imbalances.

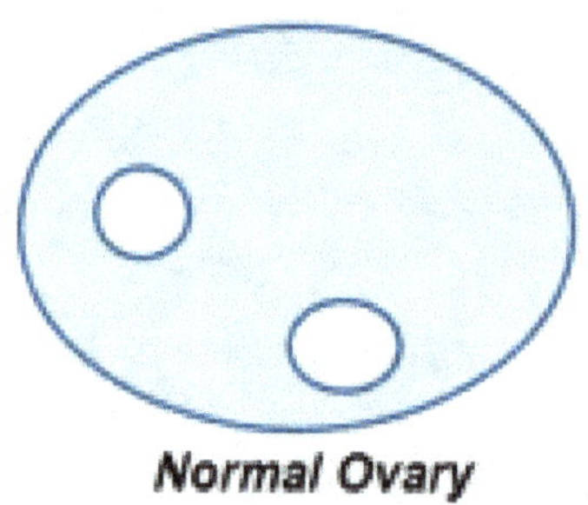

Normal Ovary

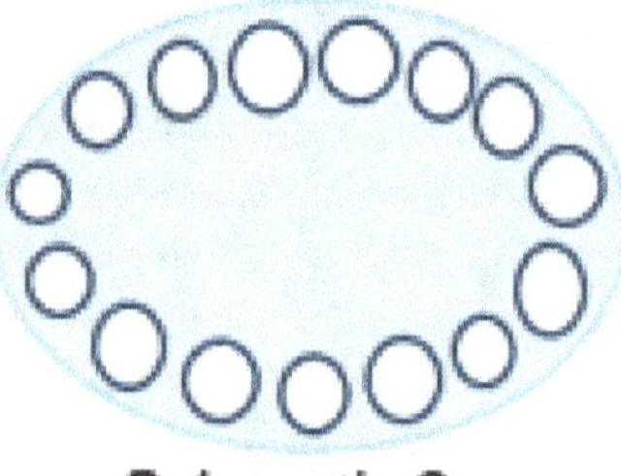

Polycystic Ovary

DIFFERENCE BETWEEN POLYCYSTIC OVARY AND POLYCYSTIC OVARIAN SYNDROME:

FEATURES	POLYCYSTIC OVARY	POLYCYSTIC OVARIAN SYNDROME
DEFINITION	Presence of multiple small cysts on the ovaries	A hormonal imbalance causing several symptoms,

		including potentially PCO
SEVERITY	Not necessarily a medical condition	A recognized medical condition with various potential health risks
SYMPTOMS	Usually no symptoms, occasionally mild pelvic pain	Irregular or absent periods, excess hair growth, acne, weight gain, fertility issues
HORMONE LEVELS	May have slightly elevated androgen levels	Elevated androgen levels, often imbalanced FSH and LH levels
OVULATION	Typically ovulates normally	May not ovulate regularly or at all
CYST SIZE AND NUMBER	May have 12 or more small cysts (5-8mm)	May have many small cysts (2-9mm)
PREVALENCE	Affects 20-25% of women of childbearing age	Affects 8-13% of women of childbearing age
TREATMENT	Usually no treatment needed, lifestyle changes may be helpful	Requires treatment to manage symptoms and reduce risks, depending on individual needs
LONG-TERM RISKS	Not associated with long-term health risks	Can increase risk of type 2 diabetes,

heart disease, and
endometrial cancer

As you can see, the main difference between PCO and PCOS is that PCOS is a hormonal imbalance that can cause a variety of symptoms, while PCO is simply the presence of multiple small cysts on the ovaries. PCO is not necessarily a medical condition, and many women with PCO have no symptoms. However, PCOS can lead to health problems.

SYMPTOMS

PCOS symptoms can be different for each woman and might show up in various ways. They can also change over time. So, if you have PCOS, your experience might not be the same as someone else with PCOS. The usual signs of PCOS include

1. Navigating Emotions with PCOS

Having PCOS might bring about emotional challenges like depression, anxiety, irritability, and mood swings. It might feel a bit like premenstrual syndrome (PMS), but the difference is that these feelings aren't limited to just before your period.

These emotional symptoms in PCOS could be because of:

✓ ***Hormone imbalances:*** *PCOS messes with your hormones, and that can affect how you feel.*
✓ ***Dealing with upsetting PCOS symptoms:*** *The physical challenges from PCOS can also take a toll on your emotions.*
✓ ***Stress from having a long-term health condition:*** *Living with a condition like PCOS can be stressful in itself.*

Another emotional effect of PCOS is a tendency towards eating disorders. Abnormal eating behaviors like binge eating and bulimia are more common in PCOS compared to the general population. While 1% of women in the general population have bulimia, it's 6% among women with PCOS. Understanding and managing these emotional aspects are crucial for overall well-being with PCOS.

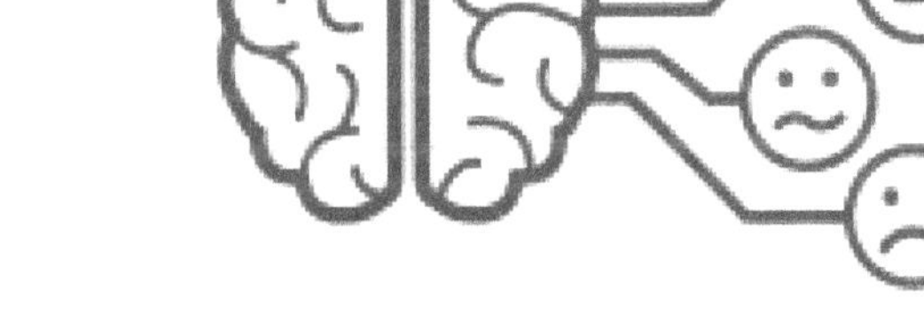

2. Insulin Resistance

If you have PCOS, you might hear about something called "insulin resistance." It's not something you can see, but it can lead to problems like diabetes and heart disease later on. Insulin resistance is quite common in PCOS, especially if you gain weight.

Now, insulin is a helpful hormone that helps your cells use sugar for energy. When you are insulin resistant, your muscles don't respond well to insulin, so your body has to produce more insulin to make it work. This can lead to feeling tired and lacking energy. Also, because your cells can't use the sugar properly, your blood sugar levels go up, and that can lead to type 2 diabetes. Type 2 diabetes can be a sneaky problem because you might not notice the symptoms for a long time. Insulin resistance also messes with the fats in your blood, raising bad cholesterol levels and increasing the chance of heart disease or a stroke.

Insulin resistance is the main reason behind many PCOS symptoms. When you have it, your body can't use insulin properly, so your pancreas has to make even more. High insulin levels mean:

✓ *You gain more weight because your body stores more fat.*

✓ *Your ovaries make more testosterone, messing up your reproductive hormones. This can make your menstrual cycle irregular or even stop your periods.*

✓ *Extra testosterone can cause acne and hirsutism (excess hair growth).*

So, managing insulin resistance is key to feeling better with PCOS.

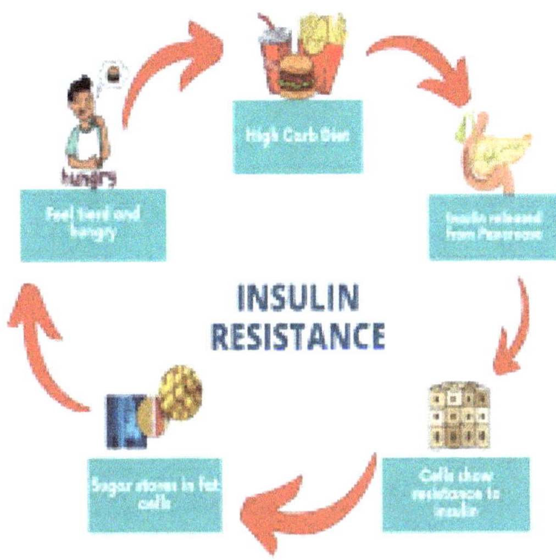

3. Fertility Problem

Having trouble getting pregnant could be one of the reasons you found out you have PCOS. When your ovaries don't release an egg, it's hard to conceive. This happens because the hormones needed to make an egg ready for release are not at the right levels.

Infertility, which means having difficulty getting pregnant, often occurs when PCOS gets more serious. In fact, about 90-95% of women who have trouble ovulating and go to fertility clinics have PCOS.

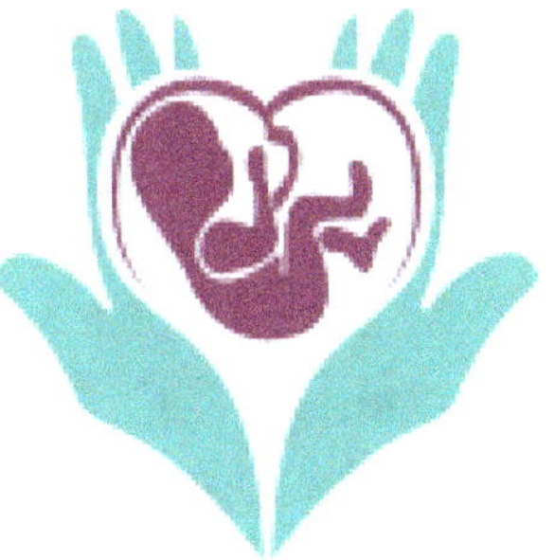

4. Period Disruption:

One noticeable effect is on your periods:

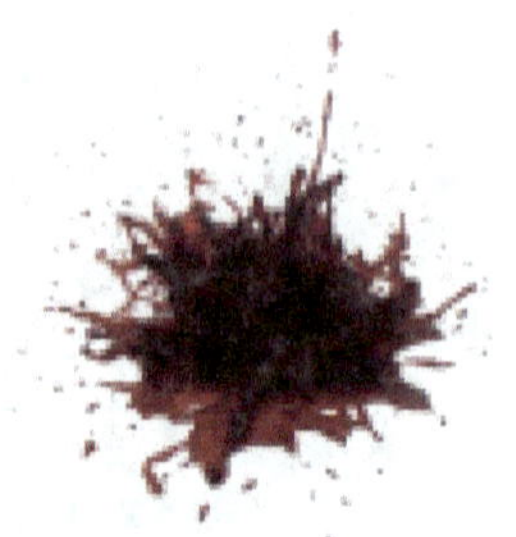

- ✓ *No Period at All (Amenorrhea):* Some with PCOS don't get their periods.
- ✓ *Irregular Periods (Oligomenorrhea):* For others, periods can be unpredictable.
- ✓ *Heavy Periods (Menorrhagia):* Periods might be heavier than usual.
- ✓ *Long-lasting Periods:* Some may experience periods that seem to go on forever.

If you have PCOS, you might have higher levels of male hormones, especially testosterone, which can lead to these period issues. But here's a silver lining — about 1 in 5 women with PCOS have normal menstrual cycles. So, while PCOS can bring challenges, there's hope that things can get better with the right guidance.

5. Weight Gain:

Having PCOS doesn't mean you're guaranteed to be overweight — it's a 50/50 chance (so, a 50% chance of being overweight and a 50% chance of not being overweight!). The main reasons for weight gain in PCOS are insulin resistance and higher levels of male hormones. This weight gain often shows up around the

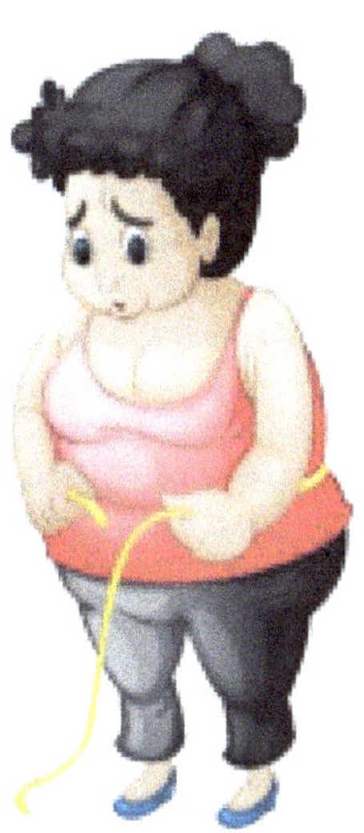

middle, like a "beer belly". When you eat carbs, your blood sugar goes up, and the pancreas releases insulin to help your body's cells absorb the sugar. But if you have insulin resistance (common in PCOS), too much sugar stays in your blood because it can't get into your cells properly. This extra sugar eventually turns into excess body fat, particularly around the belly. So, managing these factors is essential for maintaining a healthy weight with PCOS.

6. Different Hair Patterns

PCOS can affect your hair in two different ways:

Hirsutism:

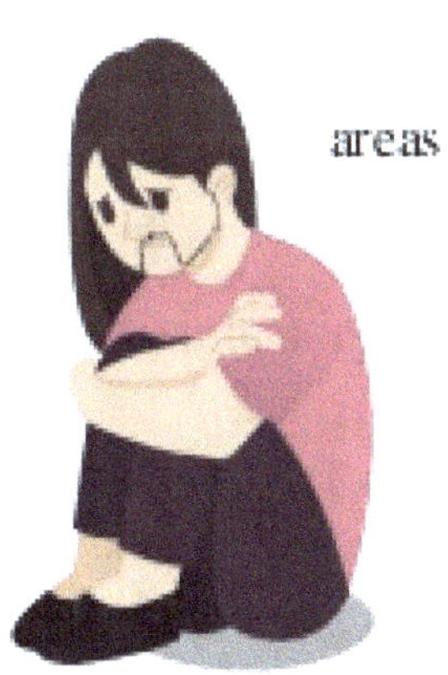

This refers to excess hair growth in areas where women typically don't have much hair, like the face, chest, stomach, and back. Think darker, thicker hair compared to the usual fine, light fuzz. It's caused by higher levels of male hormones in your body.

Alopecia or Hair Loss:

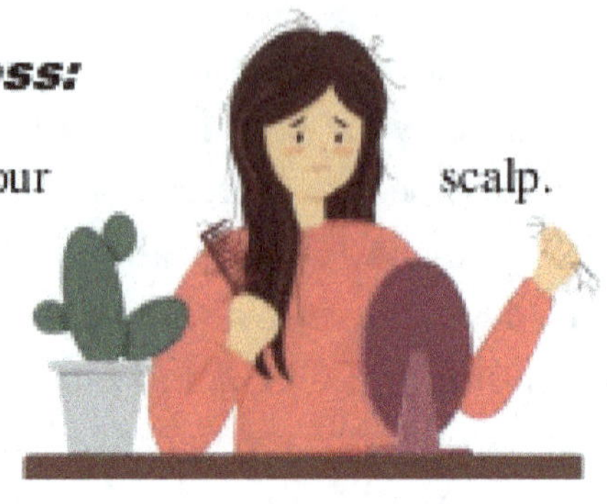

This means hair loss on your scalp. With PCOS, you might experience gradual thinning, especially around the temples or crown of your head. This can make your hair appear less dense and see-through in certain light. Don't worry, complete baldness is very rare!

7. Fatigue

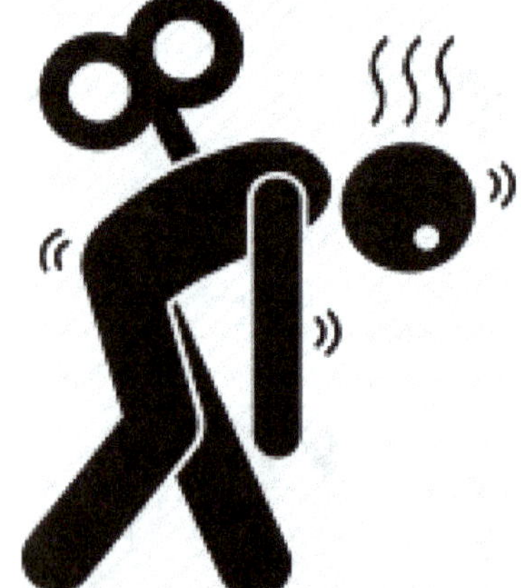

Feeling tired all the time is a common thing with PCOS. You might notice you need more sleep than before and even feel like taking a nap during the day. Waking up in the morning could be a real struggle too.

PCOS can mess with your sleep, making it harder for you to get a good night's rest. If this keeps happening, it might lead to chronic fatigue, which is feeling tired all the time. But the good news is that if you deal with these symptoms early on, you can prevent it from getting worse.

The reason behind this tiredness in PCOS is linked to insulin resistance. When you have PCOS, your body doesn't use carbohydrates properly for energy; instead, it turns them into fat. So, as you gain more weight, you also feel more and more tired. Plus, if you have PCOS, your blood sugar levels can drop really low while you sleep, making you feel exhausted the next day. Managing these factors is crucial to boost your energy levels

8. Pain:

PCOS doesn't usually cause the intense pelvic pain you might associate with big ovarian cysts. However, you might feel some discomfort in your pelvic area from time to time. This could be because of how hormones affect blood flow in the pelvic veins.

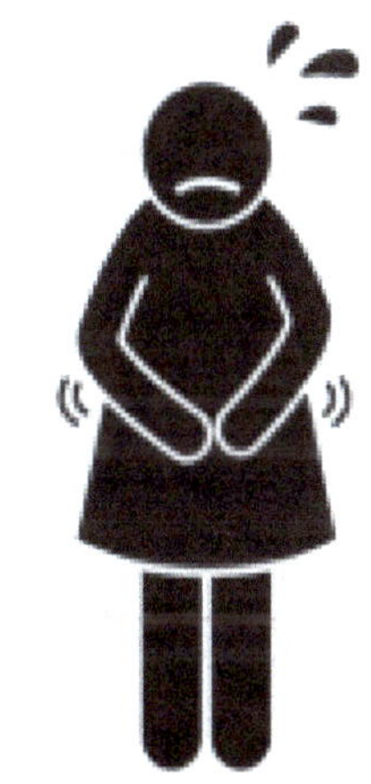

9. Skin Changes:

With PCOS, you might notice small pieces of skin called skin tags appearing on your neck or armpits. Darkened areas of skin

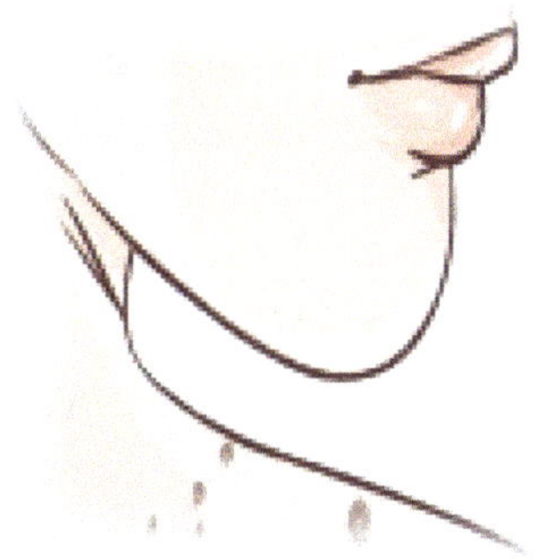

might also show up on the back of your neck, in the armpits, or under the breasts. Doctors call this condition 'acanthosis nigricans.'

10. Acne and Oily Skin:

When your male hormone levels (androgens) are high, you might get acne on your face, chest, or back. Your skin's oil-making glands work overtime, producing too much of an oily substance called sebum, and that can lead to acne.

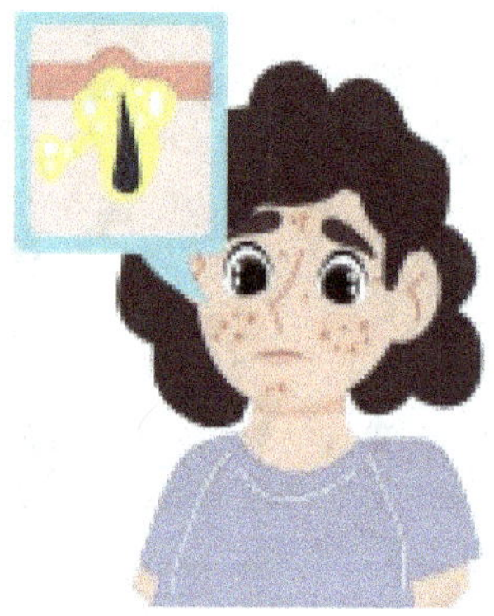

11. Depression

Depression is a symptom that often goes unnoticed with PCOS. It's more likely to happen if you have severe symptoms of PCOS. While depression can be caused by many things, PCOS might be one of them, especially if you're experiencing other PCOS symptoms.

Experts aren't sure if PCOS directly causes depression or if symptoms like weight gain trigger it. But either way, it can create a cycle where depression makes it harder to deal with PCOS symptoms, which then worsen depression.

If you notice any of these signs of depression, it's important to talk to your doctor:

1. Feeling sad for no reason for several days in a row.
2. Avoiding social activities and preferring to stay alone.
3. Crying often without a clear cause.
4. Having trouble sleeping regularly.
5. Being very hard on yourself.
6. Having thoughts of hurting yourself.

Depression can also be a side effect of medications used to treat PCOS. If you're feeling depressed, talk to your doctor. They might be able to find different medications that won't make you feel this way.

PCOS THROUGH LIFE'S CHANGES

LIFE STAGES	COMMON PCOS SYMPTOMS
ADOLESCENCE: (FIRST PERIOD ONWARDS)	• Irregular or Absent Periods • Acne • Excess Hair Growth
YOUNG ADULTHOOD: (20S-30S)	• Fertility Concerns • Weight Management • Emotional Impact
PREGNANCY:	• Increased Risk of Gestational Diabetes • Miscarriage Risk • Difficulty Getting Pregnant
PERIMENOPAUSE: (40S-50S)	• Worsening Period Irregularity • Increased Risk of Type 2 Diabetes

and Heart Disease
Emotional Changes

23

POST-
MENOPAUSE:

- Increased Risk of Endometrial Cancer
- Ongoing Weight Management
- Emotional Adjustments

CHAPTER 2:

HAIR & PCOS CONNECTION

1. Hair Composition
2. Why does hair grow or not grow?
3. Hair Growth Cycle
4. Types of Hair
5. PCOS Connection with Hair Issues
6. Hyperandrogenism
7. Connection between Hyperandrogenism and PCOS
8. Types of Hair Issues

- Hirsutism
- Androgenic Alopecia
- Hair Quality changes in PCOS

HAIR COMPOSITION

Hair, whether on your head or body, shares a similar basic composition across individuals, although there are some key differences between head and body hair:

Common Components:

Keratin:

This protein makes up around 95% of your hair. It gives hair its strength, structure, and waterproof qualities.

Melanin:

This pigment determines your hair color. Different types and amounts of melanin are responsible for blonde, brown, black, red, and gray hair.

Lipids:

Fats like sebum coat and protect your hair from damage.

Trace mineral:

Small amounts of minerals like zinc, iron, and copper contribute to hair health.

Why does hair grow or not grow?

Hair is made of a protein called keratin. Each hair strand grows longer over several months as keratin is released into the hair's root. Hair grows from something called a follicle, which is like its home. Every follicle has its own growth cycle. For example, the follicles on your scalp might grow for two to five years, while those on your hands might only grow for two months. Eventually, the growth phase stops, and then the hair falls out. After a short rest, the follicle grows another hair. Inside the follicle, there are receptors for male and female hormones, as well as enzymes that help make these hormones

HAIR GROWTH CYCLE

The hair growth cycle is how your hair grows, falls out, and grows again. It happens in three stages: growth, transition, and resting. Knowing about this cycle helps us understand how our hair grows and how conditions like PCOS can affect it. Now, let's look at each stage of the hair growth cycle:

STAGES	**DESCRIPTION**	**PCOS IMPACT**
ANAGEN PHASE (GROWTH PHASE)	Active phase of hair growth	PCOS can prolong this phase, leading to excessive or unwanted hair growth (hirsutism)
CATAGEN PHASE (TRANSITION PHASE)	Transition phase where hair stops growing	PCOS may not directly impact this phase
TELOGEN PHASE (RESTING PHASE)	Resting phase where old hair sheds and new hair begins to grow	PCOS can shorten this phase, leading to hair loss or thinning (androgenic alopecia)

PCOS can disrupt the normal balance of hormones, including androgens (male hormones), which can affect the hair growth cycle by prolonging the growth phase (anagen), shortening the resting phase (telogen), or both. This disruption can lead to excessive hair growth (hirsutism) in certain areas and hair loss or thinning on the scalp.

<u>TYPES OF HAIR</u>

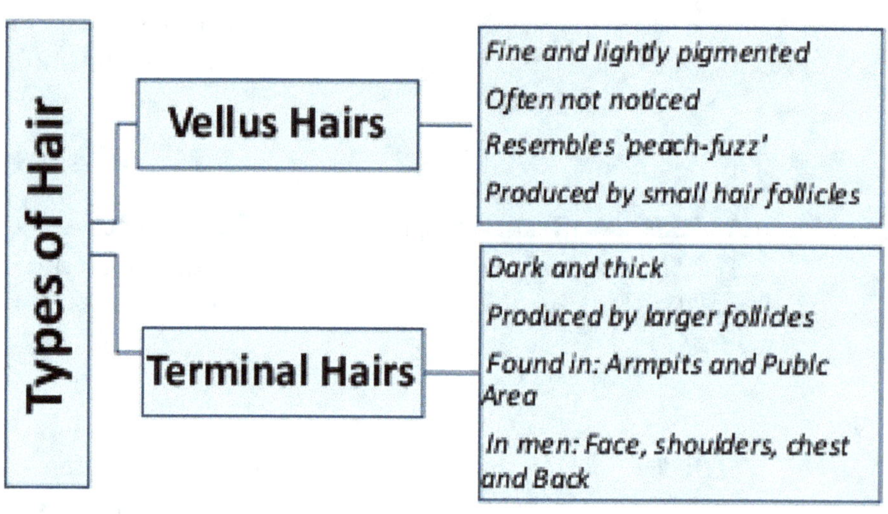

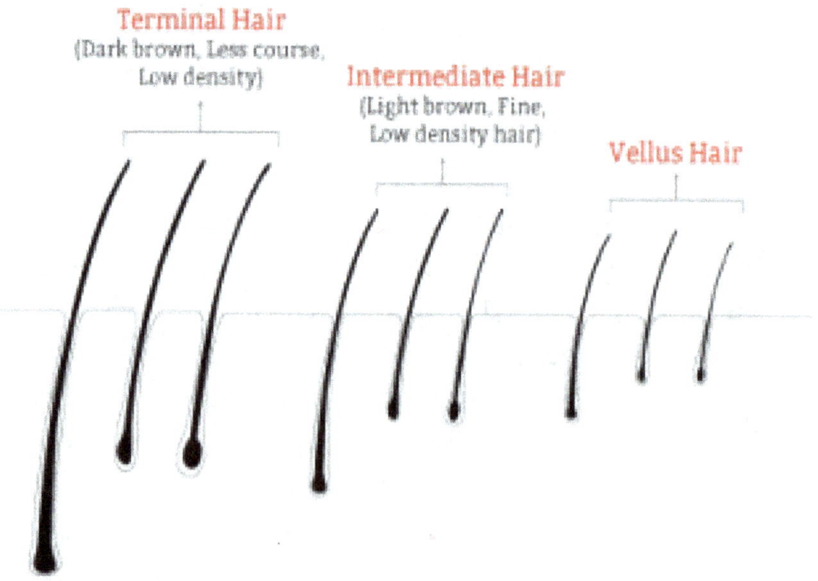

<u>PCOS CONNECTION WITH HAIR ISSUES:</u>

One big way PCOS can affect you is with your hair. Because of certain hormone imbalances, people with PCOS might notice changes in their hair, like more hair growth in places you don't want it (like on your face or chest) or less hair on your head. These changes can be frustrating and affect how you feel about yourself. Understanding this connection between PCOS and hair problems is important for finding ways to manage and cope with these changes.

<u>HYPERANDROGENISM</u>

Hyperandrogenism is a condition characterized by excessive levels of male hormones (androgens) in the body. While androgens are naturally present in both men and women, they are typically found in much higher levels in men. However, in women, elevated androgen levels can result in a variety of symptoms, including:

1. ***Hirsutism:*** *Excessive hair growth on the face, chest, back, or abdomen.*
2. ***Acne:*** *Oily skin and breakouts.*
3. ***Male pattern baldness:*** *Hair loss on the scalp.*

4. ***Irregular menstrual cycles:*** *Missed or infrequent periods.*
5. ***Deepening of the voice:*** *Less common.*
6. ***Increased muscle mass:*** *Less common.*

Connection between hyperandrogenism and PCOS:

Hyperandrogenism, which means having too many male hormones, is a key part of PCOS. Usually, in PCOS, the ovaries are the main reason for making too many male hormones. They can either produce too much male hormone on their own or be extra sensitive to the ones already in the body. Sometimes, PCOS can also happen because of issues with the adrenal glands, which also make male hormones

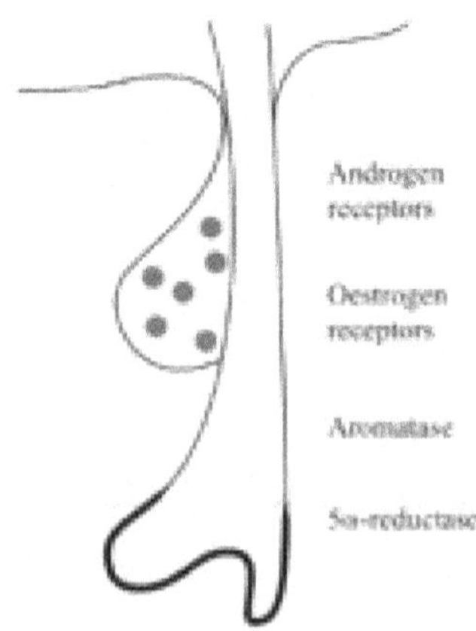

TYPES OF HAIR ISSUES IN PCOS

PCOS and its hormonal imbalances can manifest in various hair issues, impacting women's self-esteem and well-being. Here's a breakdown of three common types:

1. HIRSUTISM

Many women with PCOS worry about hirsutism, which means having too much dark and rough hair in places where men usually have it. This extra hair can show up on the face, chest, belly, back, thighs, and even around the nipples. It can be upsetting, but knowing why it happens and what you can do about it can help you handle it better.

What causes hirsutism?

The main reason for excess hair growth (hirsutism) in PCOS is having too many male hormones, like testosterone, which is called hyperandrogenism. Usually, women's bodies naturally make a little bit of these male hormones, along with the main female hormone, estrogen. But in PCOS, the balance can get messed up, causing the male hormones to increase.

How does testosterone affect hair growth?

When testosterone, a male hormone, goes up in your body, it attaches to receptors in your hair follicles. These receptors are like little switches that can turn on hair growth. When testosterone binds to these receptors, especially in certain areas, it can make hair grow thicker and darker in places where you usually don't have much hair.

2. ANDROGENIC ALOPECIA

Androgenic alopecia, also called female pattern hair loss, is a common worry for women with PCOS. It makes your hair slowly get thinner, mostly at the top and front of your head. Understanding why it happens and what you can do about it can help you feel more in control.

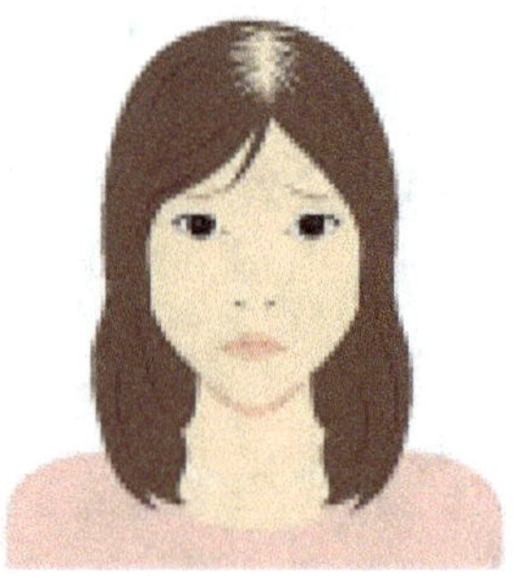

What Causes Androgenic Alopecia in PCOS?

Androgenic alopecia in PCOS happens because of too many male hormones, just like with hirsutism. These hormones mess up the normal hair growth cycle:

- **Shortened Anagen Phase *(Hair Growth Gets Shorter)*:** The active growth phase of hair (called anagen phase) gets shorter because of the male hormones. This means your hair doesn't grow as long or as thick as it should.

- **Prolonged Telogen Phase *(More Hair Falls Out)*:** The resting phase of hair (called telogen phase) gets longer because of the male hormones. This makes more hair fall out, making your hair look thinner.

What Does Androgenic Alopecia Look Like?

Androgenic alopecia can look different for everyone, but some common signs include:

- *Your hair slowly gets thinner on top of your head, especially around the crown and front.*
- *You notice more hair falling out, either on your brush or when you're styling your hair.*
- *The part in your hair looks wider.*
- *When you lift your hair, you can see more of your scalp in certain spots.*

3. HAIR QUALITY CHANGES IN PCOS:

When you have PCOS, it can affect your hair in different ways. We often hear about too much hair growth (hirsutism) or hair loss (alopecia), but changes in hair quality are also common.

What Happens to Your Hair in PCOS?

1. **Dry and Brittle Hair:** With PCOS, your body might not make enough natural oil (sebum) to keep your hair moisturized. This can make your hair feel dry, fragile, and prone to breaking.

2. **Thinner Strands**: PCOS can make your hair follicles smaller, resulting in

thinner, weaker hair that lacks volume and bounce.

3. **Dull and Faded Color:** Hormonal changes in PCOS might affect how much color pigment your hair has, leading to duller hair color and even premature graying.

4. **More Frizz and Tangles:** Because your hair is dry and not as smooth, it can become frizzy and tangled more easily, making it harder to manage.

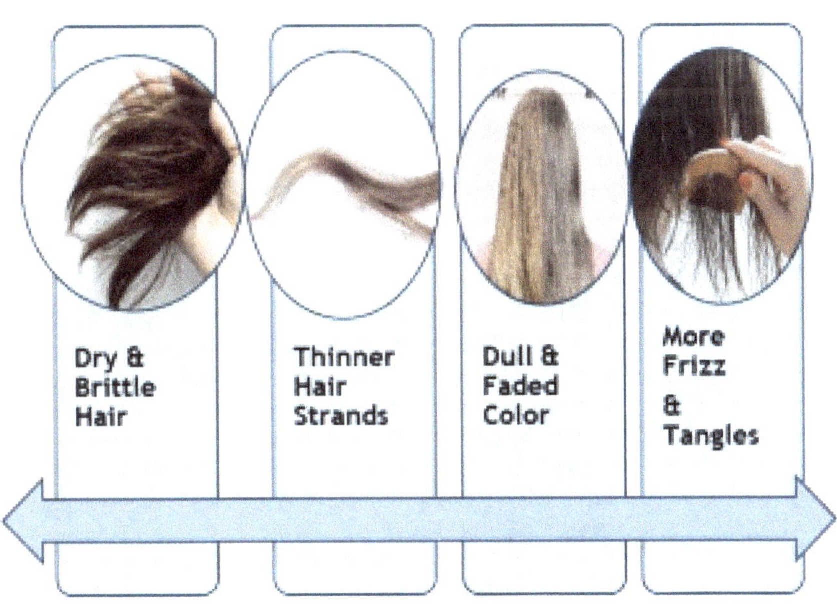

CHAPTER 3:

NAVIGATING HORMONAL IMBALANCES

1. Hormones
2. Types of hormones
3. Hormonal Shifts in PCOS
4. Causes of Hormonal Imbalances in PCOS
   - Genetic Factor
   - Lifestyle Factor
   - Environmental Factors
   - Medical Conditions and Medications
5. Diagnostic Test for Hormonal Imbalances
   - Blood Test
   - Saliva Test
   - Urine Test
   - Ultrasound
6. Interpreting Test Results

HORMONES

Hormones are like the invisible messengers of your body, constantly sending signals to different organs and tissues, telling them what to do and when. These powerful chemicals play a crucial role in virtually every bodily function.

They help with things like making us grow, keeping us healthy, and controlling our moods and sleep. Hormones also make sure our body stays balanced, even when things around us change. They can tell our cells what to do, like releasing other hormones or turning genes on and off. So basically, hormones are like little messengers that keep everything in our body working smoothly.

TYPES OF HORMONE

There are over 50 different types of hormones, each with a unique role. Some key hormones include:

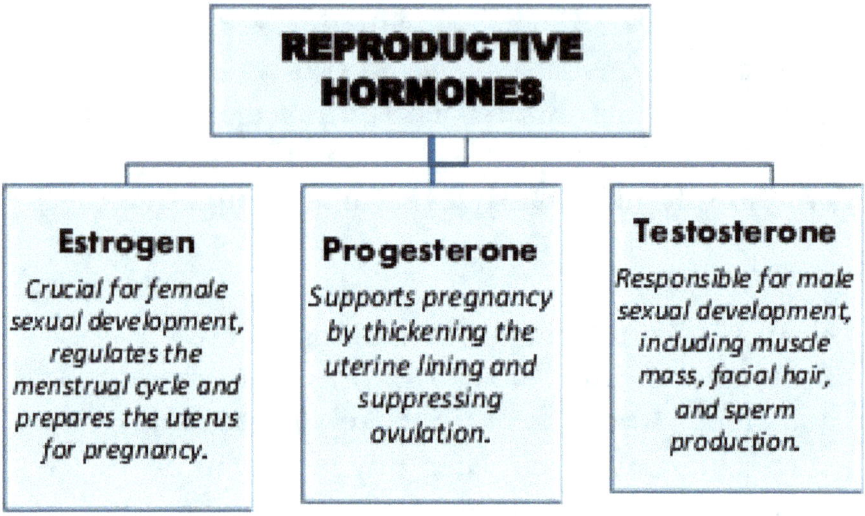

REPRODUCTIVE HORMONES

Estrogen

Crucial for female sexual development, regulates the menstrual cycle and prepares the uterus for pregnancy.

Progesterone

Supports pregnancy by thickening the uterine lining and suppressing ovulation.

Testosterone

Responsible for male sexual development, including muscle mass, facial hair, and sperm production.

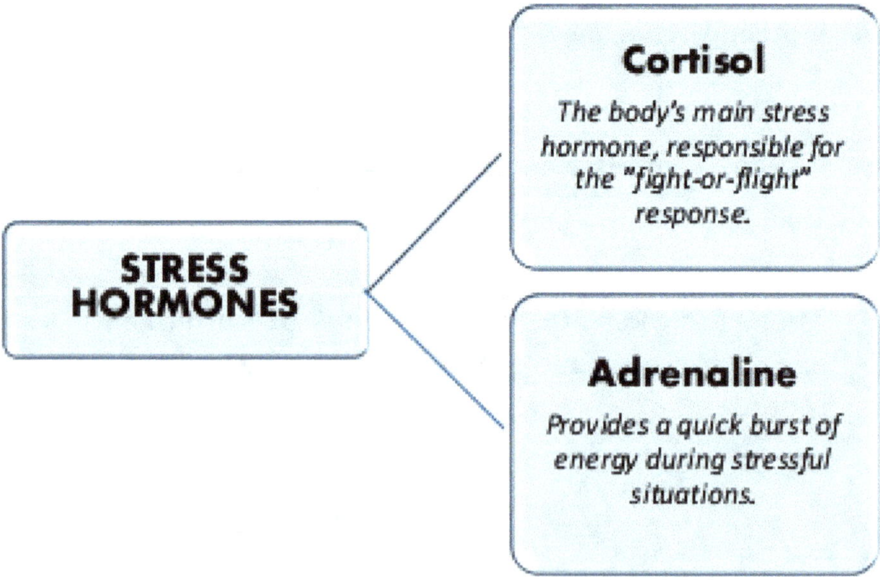

STRESS HORMONES

Cortisol

The body's main stress hormone, responsible for the "fight-or-flight" response.

Adrenaline

Provides a quick burst of energy during stressful situations.

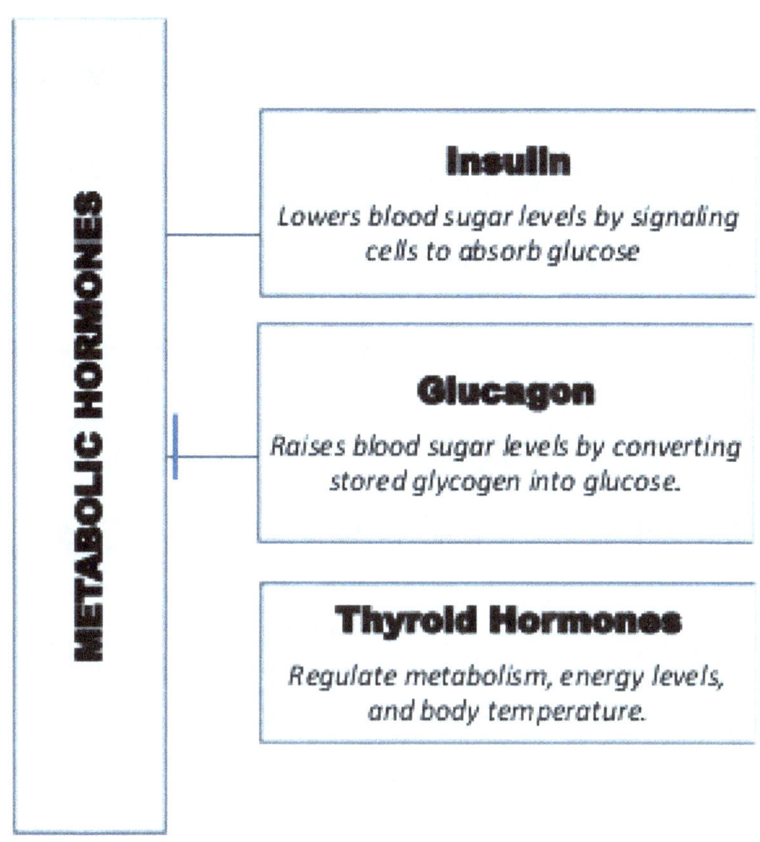

HORMONAL SHIFTS IN PCOS

Hormone	Function in healthy individuals	Pcos-related changes
Estrogen	Regulates menstrual cycle, bone health, mood	↑ Elevated estradiol, ↓ decreased SHBG (binding protein)

Hormone	Function	PCOS Level
Progesterone	Supports pregnancy, balances estrogen effects	↓ Deficiency during ovulation, irregular levels
Testosterone	Male sexual development, muscle mass	↑ Elevated free and total testosterone
Insulin	Regulates blood sugar	↑ Insulin resistance, high blood sugar (hyperglycemia)
Glucagon	Raises blood sugar	↑↓ Normal to slightly elevated
Thyroid hormones (T3, T4)	Regulate metabolism, energy levels	↔ Normal to slightly abnormal levels, but thyroid issues can co-occur with PCOS
Cortisol	Stress hormone	↑ Elevated in some individuals with PCOS due to stress and inflammation
Adrenaline	Fight-or-flight response	↔ Similar to healthy individuals, but stress response may be amplified in PCOS

PCOS can cause disruptions in hormone levels, leading to higher levels of testosterone, insulin, cortisol, and adrenaline, while also affecting estrogen, progesterone, glucagon, and thyroid hormones. These imbalances contribute to the symptoms and complications associated with

PCOS, such as irregular periods, infertility, weight gain, and hirsutism.

CAUSES OF HORMONAL IMBALANCES IN PCOS

Understanding why hormonal imbalances occur in PCOS is crucial for managing the condition effectively. The hormonal imbalances associated with PCOS can be influenced by several factors, including genetics, lifestyle choices, environmental factors, and certain medical conditions or medications.

Causes of Hormonal Imbalances in PCOS:

Genetic Factors:

PCOS tends to run in families, suggesting that genetics play a role. Some people may inherit genes that make them more likely to develop hormonal imbalances, insulin resistance, and irregular ovulation, which are key features of PCOS.

Lifestyle Factors:

Our daily habits can also impact hormone levels in PCOS:

1. *Diet*: Eating too many sugary or refined foods can make insulin resistance worse, which affects hormone levels.
2. *Exercise:* Not getting enough physical activity can also worsen insulin resistance and hormonal imbalances
3. *Stress:* Feeling stressed all the time can mess with hormones like cortisol and adrenaline, which can make PCOS symptoms worse.
4. *Sleep:* Not getting good sleep can throw off your hormones, especially insulin and sex hormones.

Environmental Factors:

Stuff in our environment can mess with our hormones too. Chemicals found in things like plastics and pesticides can interfere with our hormones, making PCOS symptoms worse.

Medical Conditions and Medications:

Sometimes, other health problems or medicines can affect our hormones and make PCOS symptoms worse:

1. **Thyroid Problems (Hypothyroidism):** If your thyroid isn't working right, it can mess with your hormones and make PCOS symptoms worse.
2. **Too Much Prolactin (Hyperprolactinemia):** Having too much of a hormone called prolactin can mess with ovulation and periods, making PCOS symptoms worse.
3. **Medicines:** Some medicines, like certain birth control pills or steroids, can also affect our hormones and make PCOS symptoms worse.

By understanding these factors, people with PCOS can make changes in their lives to help manage their symptoms and feel better overall.

DIAGNOSTIC TESTS FOR HORMONAL IMBALANCES IN PCOS

Diagnosing hormonal imbalances, particularly in conditions like Polycystic Ovary Syndrome (PCOS), requires a thorough understanding of the various diagnostic tests available. This guide aims to provide detailed explanations of these tests, including blood tests, saliva tests, urine tests, and ultrasound, as well as how to interpret the results to gain insights into your health.

Blood Tests:

Hormone Panel:
A comprehensive blood test that measures levels of various hormones including estrogen, progesterone, testosterone, insulin, cortisol, thyroid hormones, and others. Elevated testosterone and insulin levels, along with imbalances in other hormones, can indicate PCOS

Glucose Tolerance Test (GTT):
Evaluates how your body processes glucose. Insulin resistance, a common feature of PCOS, can be detected through this test.

Lipid Profile:
Assesses cholesterol levels which may be abnormal in PCOS due to insulin resistance.

Saliva Tests:

Cortisol Saliva Test:

Measures cortisol levels throughout the day, providing insights into adrenal function and stress response, which can be disrupted in PCOS

Sex Hormone Saliva Test:
Evaluates levels of sex hormones like estrogen, progesterone, and testosterone, offering a non-invasive way to monitor hormonal balance.

Urine Tests:

Urine Hormone Metabolites:
Assess the breakdown products of hormones, offering insights into hormone metabolism and potential imbalances.

Ultrasound:

Pelvic Ultrasound:
Visualizes the ovaries to detect cysts, a common feature of PCOS. It also assesses the size and morphology of the ovaries and measures the thickness of the uterine lining.

INTERPRETING TEST RESULTS:

Consultation with Healthcare Provider:

It's crucial to discuss test results with a healthcare provider who can provide personalized interpretation based on your medical history and symptoms

Hormonal Patterns:

Understanding the interplay between different hormones and how their levels change throughout the menstrual cycle or day can provide valuable insights.

Treatment Implications:

Test results guide treatment strategies, such as lifestyle modifications, medications to regulate hormones, and management of associated conditions like insulin resistance and high cholesterol.

Monitoring Progress:

Regular monitoring through follow-up tests helps track the effectiveness of treatment and make necessary adjustments

CHAPTER 4:
TREATMENT FOR HAIR RELATED ISSUES IN PCOS

1. Pharmaceutical Interventions
   - Hormonal Contraceptives
   - Anti-Androgen Medications
   - Insulin-Sensitizing Agent
2. Tropical Treatments
   - Prescription Creams or Gels
   - Minoxidil
3. Hair Growth Treatments
   - Finasteride
   - Dutasteride
   - Oral Supplements
   - Scalp Massage for Hair Growth
   - Platelet-Rich Plasma (PRP) Therapy
   - Micro needling
   - Hair Transplant Surgery
4. Hair Removal Treatments
   - Shaving
   - Plucking
   - Waxing
   - Bleaching
   - Depilatory Creams
   - Laser Hair Removal
   - IPL (Intense Pulsed Light) Therapy
   - Electrolysis

Hair-related symptoms in PCOS are more than just a cosmetic concern; they can significantly impact a person's self-esteem and quality of life. Understanding and managing these symptoms are essential for overall well-being and confidence. From excess hair growth to hair loss, addressing these issues is crucial for individuals with PCOS to feel comfortable and confident in their bodies.

There are various treatment options available for managing hair-related symptoms in PCOS, ranging from medical interventions to holistic approaches. Medical treatments may include medications like hormonal contraceptives or anti-androgen drugs to regulate hormone levels and reduce excess hair growth. Additionally, holistic approaches such as dietary changes, supplements, and lifestyle modifications can complement medical treatments to support overall hair health. Professional treatments like laser hair removal or scalp treatments may also be considered for targeted management of specific symptoms. It's important to explore these options with a healthcare professional to create a personalized treatment plan that addresses individual needs and preferences.

<u>PHARMACUETICAL INTERVENTIONS</u>

Pharmaceutical interventions are commonly used to manage PCOS symptoms and promote hair harmony. These treatments target hormonal imbalances and aim to regulate menstrual cycles, reduce androgen levels, and improve hair growth patterns.

1. Hormonal Contraceptives:

Birth control pills containing estrogen and progestin are often prescribed to regulate menstrual cycles and reduce androgen levels in women with PCOS. These pills can help improve hirsutism (excess hair growth) and acne, but may take several months to show results.

2. Anti-Androgen Medications:

Drugs such as spironolactone and finasteride are anti-androgen medications that can block the effects of androgens (male hormones) on the hair follicles. They help reduce hirsutism and prevent hair loss in women with PCOS.

3. Insulin-Sensitizing Agents:

Metformin is a medication commonly used to improve insulin sensitivity in individuals with PCOS who have insulin resistance. By reducing insulin levels, metformin can help regulate menstrual cycles, improve ovulation, and reduce androgen levels, which may indirectly improve hair growth patterns.

It's essential to consult with a healthcare provider before starting any pharmaceutical interventions for PCOS and hair concerns. They can assess individual needs, provide personalized treatment recommendations, and monitor for any potential side effects or interactions with other medications. Additionally, pharmaceutical treatments are often used in combination with lifestyle modifications and complementary therapies to achieve optimal results in managing PCOS symptoms and promoting hair harmony.

TOPICAL TREATMENTS:

Topical medications, such as topical anti-androgens or minoxidil (Rogaine), can be applied directly to the scalp to promote hair growth and prevent further hair loss in

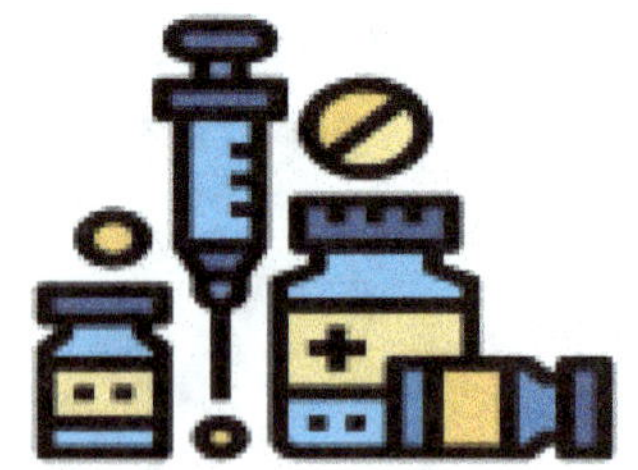

individuals with PCOS-related alopecia (hair loss).

PRESCRIPTION CREAMS OR GELS

Prescription creams or gels are topical treatments that are applied directly to the skin to address specific concerns, such as excessive hair growth or hair loss, often associated with conditions like PCOS. These creams or gels may contain active ingredients like eflornithine hydrochloride, which can slow down the growth of unwanted facial hair (hirsutism) in women with PCOS. Alternatively, topical corticosteroids may be prescribed to reduce inflammation and itching associated with scalp conditions, such as alopecia areata or seborrheic dermatitis. It's essential to follow the instructions provided by your healthcare provider and use these prescription creams or gels as directed for optimal results.

Minoxidil

Minoxidil is a medication commonly used to treat hair loss (alopecia) and promote hair regrowth in conditions like PCOS. It comes in the form of a topical solution or foam that is applied directly to the scalp. Minoxidil works by widening the blood vessels in the scalp, increasing blood flow to the hair follicles, and stimulating hair growth. While the exact mechanism of action is not fully understood, minoxidil is believed to prolong the growth phase of

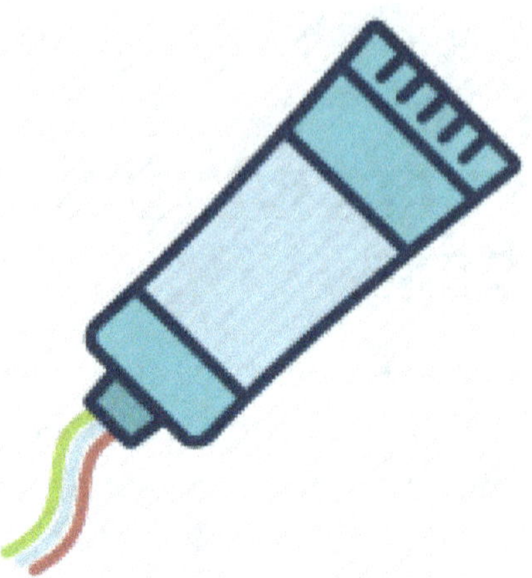

the hair cycle (anagen phase) and shorten the resting phase (telogen phase), leading to thicker, longer, and more robust hair. It's important to note that results may vary from person to person, and consistent use of minoxidil as directed by a healthcare provider is necessary to see improvements in hair density and thickness. Additionally, it's essential to be patient, as it may take several months of continuous use before noticeable results are achieved.

HAIR GROWTH TREATMENTS

Finasteride and Dutasteride can be used as hair growth treatments in individuals with PCOS experiencing hair thinning or alopecia. These medications work by targeting the hormonal imbalances associated with PCOS, particularly the elevated levels of androgens like testosterone and DHT. By reducing the effects of these hormones on the hair follicles, Finasteride and Dutasteride can help promote hair regrowth and improve overall hair health in individuals with PCOS. However, it's important to consult with a healthcare professional before starting any hair growth treatment to ensure it's safe and appropriate for your individual needs, especially considering the potential side effects.

Finasteride:

Finasteride is a medication that's commonly used to treat hair loss, especially in men. It works by blocking the conversion of testosterone into dihydrotestosterone (DHT), a hormone that can contribute to hair thinning and baldness. By reducing DHT levels, finasteride helps to slow down hair loss and promote hair regrowth. It's taken orally in the form of a pill and is usually prescribed by a doctor. While finasteride can be effective for treating male pattern baldness, its use in women, especially those with PCOS, may be limited due to potential side effects and safety concerns.

Dutasteride:

Dutasteride is another medication used for treating hair loss, particularly in men with male pattern baldness. Like finasteride, dutasteride works by inhibiting the conversion of testosterone into DHT. However, dutasteride is more potent and has a longer half-life 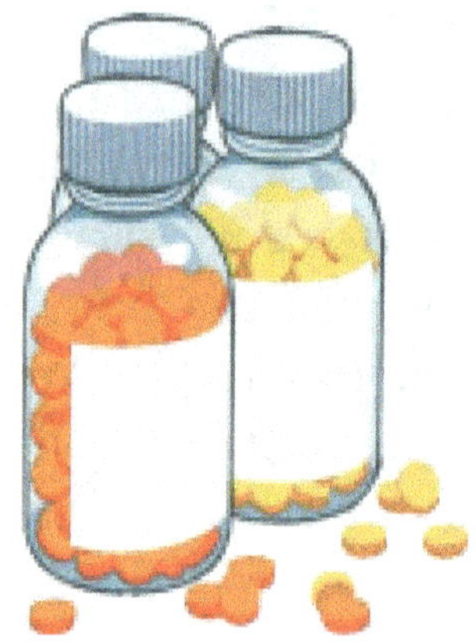 compared to finasteride, meaning it may be more effective in reducing DHT levels. While dutasteride is not approved by the FDA for treating hair loss, some doctors may prescribe it off-label for this purpose. As with finasteride, the use of dutasteride in women, including those with PCOS, may pose risks and should be carefully evaluated by a healthcare professional.

ORAL SUPPLEMENTS

1.Biotin:

Biotin, also known as vitamin B7, is a popular supplement for promoting hair growth. It helps in the production of keratin, a protein that makes up our hair, skin, and nails. Biotin may improve hair thickness and strength, reducing hair loss and promoting healthier hair growth. People with PCOS often experience hair-related issues like thinning or excessive hair growth, and biotin supplementation can support hair health in such cases.

2. Vitamins:

Vitamin D:

Vitamin D plays a crucial role in hair follicle cycling and can help regulate hair growth. Low levels of vitamin D have been linked to hair loss, so ensuring adequate vitamin D intake is important for maintaining healthy hair. Individuals with PCOS may have a higher risk of vitamin D deficiency, making supplementation particularly beneficial for them.

Vitamin E:

Vitamin E is an antioxidant that helps protect cells, including those in hair follicles, from damage caused by free radicals. It promotes blood circulation to the scalp, which can enhance hair growth and prevent hair loss. Vitamin E supplementation may benefit individuals with PCOS by supporting overall hair health and reducing hair-related concerns.

3.Saw Palmetto:

Saw palmetto is a plant extract commonly used as a natural remedy for hair loss and promoting hair growth. It is believed to inhibit the enzyme 5-alpha-reductase, which converts testosterone into dihydrotestosterone (DHT), a hormone associated with hair loss. By blocking DHT production, saw palmetto may help prevent hair thinning and promote thicker, healthier hair growth. In individuals with PCOS, who may experience hormonal imbalances and elevated androgen levels contributing to hair issues, saw palmetto supplementation could be beneficial in restoring hair harmony.

These oral supplements offer potential benefits for individuals with PCOS seeking to improve hair health and address hair-related concerns. However, it's essential to consult with a healthcare professional before starting any new supplements, especially if you have underlying health conditions or are taking medications, to ensure safety and effectiveness. Additionally, supplements should be used as part of a comprehensive approach to hair care and management, including a balanced diet, proper hair care practices, and addressing any underlying hormonal imbalances associated with PCOS.

SCALP MASSAGE FOR HAIR GROWTH

Scalp massage is a simple and effective technique that can help promote hair growth, especially for individuals with PCOS who may experience hair thinning or loss. Here's how it works:

Increased Blood Circulation:

Massaging the scalp helps to increase blood circulation to the hair follicles. This improved blood flow delivers more oxygen and nutrients to the follicles, which can stimulate hair growth and strengthen the hair strands.

Stress Reduction:

PCOS and hormonal imbalances can lead to stress, which is known to contribute to hair problems. Scalp massage helps to relax the muscles and reduce stress levels, which in turn can improve the health of the hair follicles and promote growth.

Stimulation of Hair Follicles:

The gentle pressure applied during scalp massage can help to stimulate the hair follicles, encouraging them to produce new hair strands. This can be particularly beneficial for individuals with PCOS, as hormonal imbalances may disrupt the normal hair growth cycle.

Distribution of Natural Oils:

Scalp massage helps to distribute the natural oils produced by the scalp, known as sebum, along the hair shafts. This helps to moisturize the hair and scalp, preventing dryness and breakage, and promoting overall hair health.

To perform a scalp massage:

1. *Use your fingertips to gently massage the scalp in circular motions.*
2. *Start at the front of the scalp and work your way back, covering the entire scalp.*
3. *Apply light to moderate pressure, being careful not to tug or pull on the hair.*

4. *Massage for 5-10 minutes, focusing on areas where hair thinning or loss is most noticeable.*
5. *You can use a natural oil, such as coconut oil or almond oil, to enhance the massage and provide additional nourishment to the scalp and hair.*

Incorporating scalp massage into your regular hair care routine can be a simple yet effective way to promote hair growth and improve the overall health and appearance of your hair, especially for individuals with PCOS seeking to achieve hair harmony.

PLATELET-RICH PLASMA (PRP) THERAPY

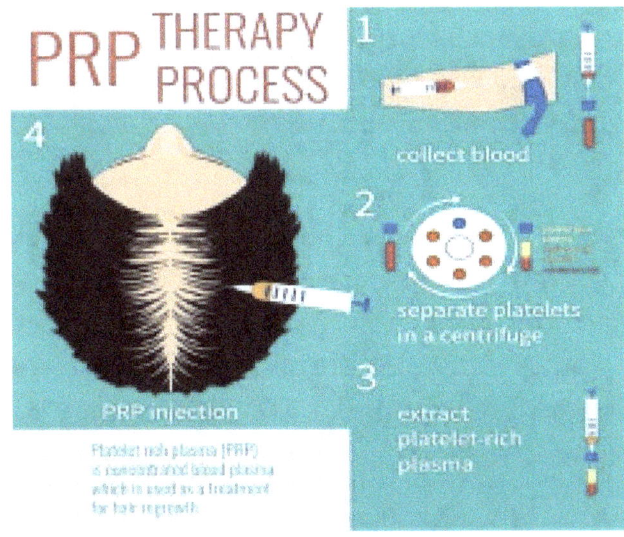

PRP Therapy involves using a concentrated form of a component found in our blood called platelets. These platelets contain growth factors and other substances that can help with tissue repair and regeneration.

During the PRP procedure, a small amount of blood is drawn from the patient, similar to getting blood drawn for a regular test. This blood is then processed to separate the platelets from the rest of the blood components. Once the platelets are isolated, they are concentrated into a small amount of plasma, forming the Platelet-Rich Plasma.

The PRP solution is then injected or applied to the scalp in areas where hair loss or thinning is a concern. The growth factors in the PRP solution stimulate the hair follicles, promoting hair growth and improving hair density.

For individuals with PCOS, PRP Therapy can be beneficial in addressing hair loss or thinning associated with hormonal imbalances. It is a minimally invasive procedure that is generally well-tolerated and can be performed in a clinical setting.

It's important to note that PRP Therapy may require multiple sessions spaced out over several weeks to months to achieve optimal results. Additionally, results may vary from person to person, and maintenance treatments may be needed to sustain the improvements in hair growth.

Overall, PRP Therapy is a promising option for individuals with PCOS looking to improve hair harmony and restore confidence in their appearance.

MICRONEEDLING

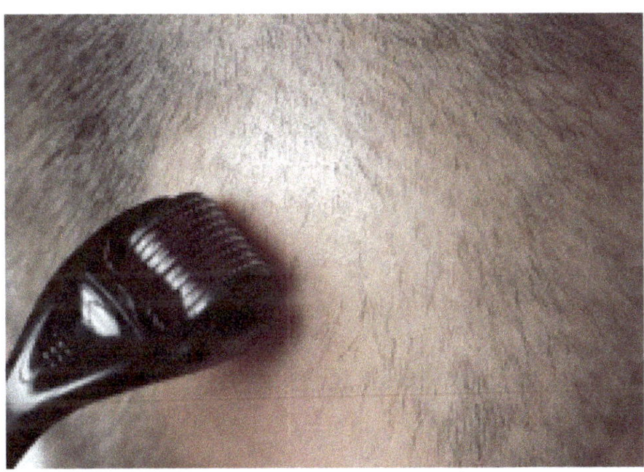

Microneedling is a procedure that involves using a device with tiny needles to create small punctures in the skin on your scalp. This process is also known as collagen induction therapy. The idea behind microneedling is to stimulate the body's natural wound healing process, which can promote hair growth.

In PCOS, hormonal imbalances can lead to changes in hair growth patterns, including excess hair growth in some areas (hirsutism) and hair

thinning or loss (alopecia) in others.
Microneedling may offer a potential solution for
addressing hair concerns associated with PCOS.

During a microneedling session, the device is
gently rolled or pressed onto the scalp, creating
microscopic injuries in the skin. These tiny
punctures stimulate the production of growth
factors and increase blood flow to the scalp,
which can nourish hair follicles and encourage
hair growth. Additionally, microneedling may
help improve the absorption of topical
treatments, such as minoxidil or hair growth
serums, by enhancing their penetration into the
scalp.

Microneedling is considered a safe and
minimally invasive procedure for promoting hair
growth, with minimal downtime and side effects.
However, it's essential to consult with a qualified
healthcare professional or dermatologist before
undergoing microneedling, especially if you have
PCOS or other underlying medical conditions.
They can assess your individual needs and
determine if microneedling is a suitable option
for you.

Microneedling may offer a promising approach
for addressing hair concerns in individuals with
PCOS by promoting hair growth and improving
overall hair health. Combined with other
treatment modalities and lifestyle interventions,
microneedling can contribute to achieving hair

harmony and enhancing self-confidence in individuals with PCOS.

HAIR TRANSPLANT SURGERY

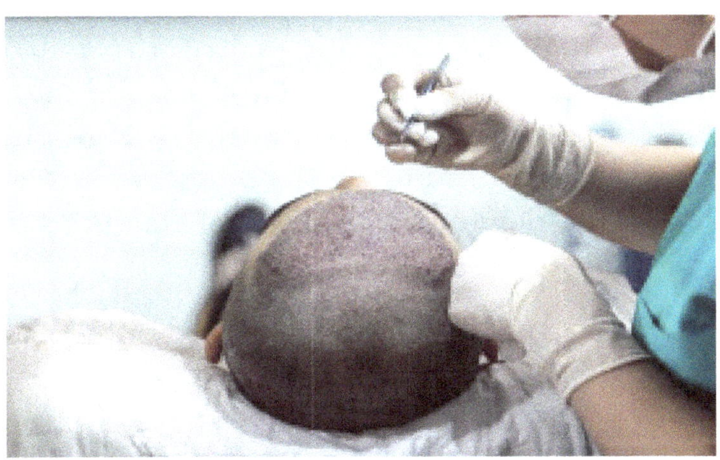

Hair transplant surgery is a procedure used to treat hair loss and restore hair growth in areas where hair is thinning or missing. Hair transplant surgery can be an option for individuals with PCOS who are experiencing significant hair loss and are looking to regain a fuller head of hair.

During a hair transplant surgery, hair follicles are taken from areas of the scalp where hair is thicker or resistant to the effects of hormones, such as the back or sides of the head. These follicles are then transplanted into the areas of the scalp where hair loss has occurred. The procedure is typically performed under local anesthesia and can take several hours to complete, depending on the extent of hair loss and the number of follicles being transplanted.

There are two main techniques used in hair transplant surgery: follicular unit transplantation (FUT) and follicular unit extraction (FUE). In FUT, a strip of skin containing hair follicles is removed from the donor area and dissected into individual follicular units for transplantation. In FUE, individual follicular units are harvested directly from the donor area using a small punch-like instrument.

After the transplant, the newly transplanted hair follicles may go through a resting phase before starting to grow new hair. It may take several months for the full results of the transplant to become apparent, as the newly transplanted hair gradually grows and blends in with the existing hair.

Hair transplant surgery can be an effective solution for individuals with PCOS who are struggling with hair loss or thinning. However, it's essential to consult with a qualified and experienced hair transplant surgeon to determine if you are a suitable candidate for the procedure and to discuss the potential risks and benefits.

<u>HAIR REMOVAL TREATMENTS</u>

Hair removal treatments can be helpful for managing excess hair growth (hirsutism) and achieving hair harmony in individuals with PCOS. Here are some options:

<u>Shaving</u>

Shaving is a common method used for hair removal, especially for women with PCOS who may experience excessive hair growth in unwanted areas. When it comes to managing hair growth in PCOS, shaving can provide a temporary solution by cutting the hair at the surface level, giving the skin a smooth appearance. It's relatively quick, easy, and can be done at home without much hassle. However, it's essential to note that shaving only removes hair from the surface, so the hair will grow back relatively quickly, usually within a few days to a week. Additionally, shaving doesn't affect the hair follicle or its growth patterns, so it doesn't provide a long-term solution for managing excessive hair growth associated with PCOS.

Plucking

Plucking is a method of hair removal where individual hairs are pulled out from the root using tweezers. When plucking hairs in PCOS, it's essential to be gentle and careful to avoid causing irritation or damage to the skin. Plucking can be effective for removing individual hairs, but it may not be practical for larger areas of hair growth. It's important to consider the time and effort required for plucking, especially if dealing with extensive hirsutism.

While plucking can provide temporary relief from unwanted hair, it's not a permanent solution. The hair will eventually grow back, and repeated plucking can lead to skin irritation, ingrown hairs, and potentially scarring. Additionally, plucking may not address the underlying hormonal imbalance causing the excess hair growth in PCOS.

Waxing

Waxing is a popular method for removing unwanted hair from different parts of the body, including the legs, arms, face, and bikini area. It involves applying a thin layer of wax onto the skin, allowing it to cool and harden, and then quickly pulling it off in the opposite direction of hair growth, removing the hair from the root.

Waxing can be both beneficial and challenging. On one hand, waxing offers a temporary solution for managing excess hair growth associated with PCOS, particularly in areas such as the face, chest, and back. Since waxing removes hair from the root, it can result in smoother skin and slower regrowth compared to shaving.

However, there are also considerations to keep in mind when waxing with PCOS. Individuals with PCOS may have more sensitive skin or be prone to ingrown hairs, which can occur when hair grows back into the skin after waxing. This can lead to irritation, redness, and even infection, especially in areas with coarse or dense hair. Additionally, hormonal fluctuations in PCOS can affect hair growth patterns, making it necessary to wax more frequently to maintain desired results. It's essential to choose a reputable salon or esthetician experienced in working with clients with PCOS and sensitive skin to minimize the risk of complications.

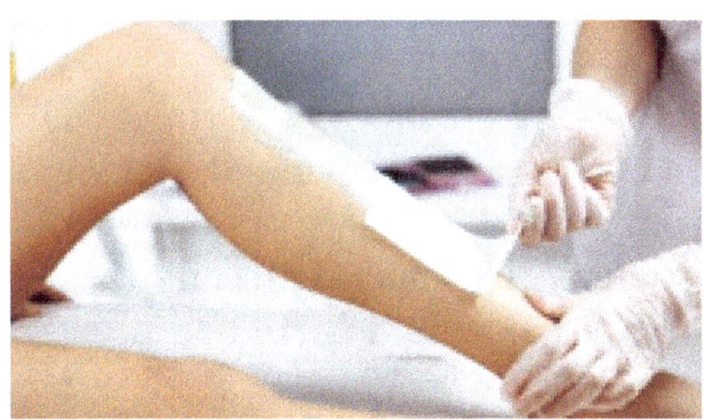

Bleaching

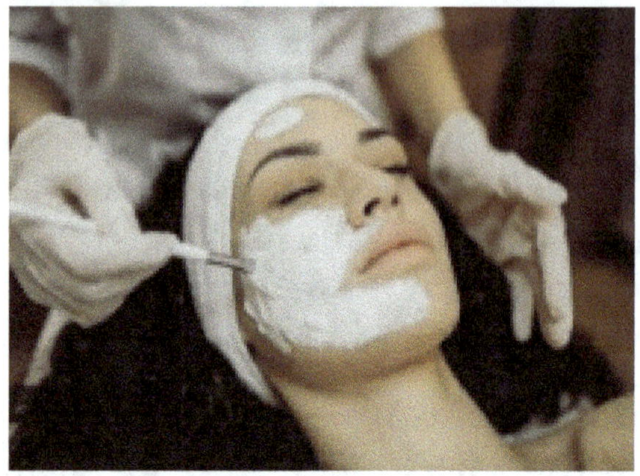

Bleaching is a method used to lighten the color of hair, making it less noticeable. In the context of PCOS (Polycystic Ovary Syndrome) and managing hair-related concerns, bleaching is often considered as a temporary solution for reducing the appearance of excess hair growth, particularly in areas affected by hirsutism.

While hirsutism can cause distress and affect self-esteem, it's essential to note that bleaching does not remove hair from the root or stop its growth. Instead, it simply changes the color of the hair, making it less noticeable against the skin.

Bleaching creams or solutions contain chemicals like hydrogen peroxide or ammonia, which work to lighten the pigment in the hair shaft. These products are applied directly to the hair and left on for a specified period before being washed off. While bleaching can be done at home, it's important to follow the instructions carefully to avoid irritation or adverse reactions, especially for individuals with sensitive skin or conditions like PCOS.

It's crucial to understand that bleaching provides only temporary relief from the appearance of excess hair growth and does not address the underlying hormonal imbalances associated with PCOS.

Depilatory Creams

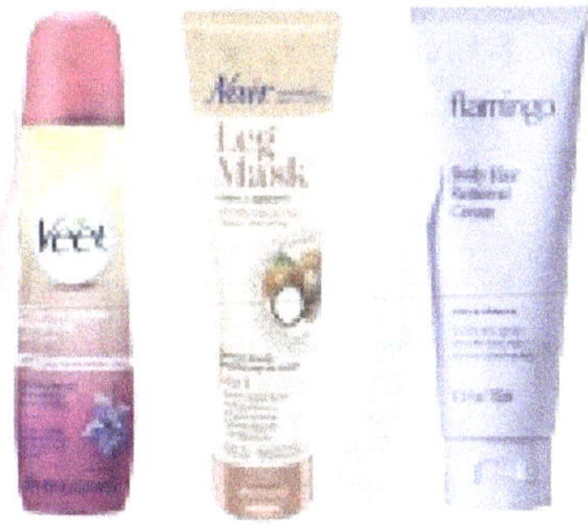

Depilatory creams are products used for removing hair from the skin's surface. They work by breaking down the protein structure of the hair, which makes it easier to wipe away. These creams are often used as an alternative to shaving or waxing because they can be less painful and quicker. Depilatory creams offer a temporary solution for removing this excess hair, providing a smoother appearance to the skin.

However, it's essential to follow the instructions carefully and perform a patch test before using these creams, as they can cause skin irritation or allergic reactions in some individuals. Additionally, depilatory creams only remove hair at the surface level, so hair will grow back relatively quickly compared to other hair removal methods like waxing or laser treatment. Therefore, regular application may be necessary to maintain hair-free skin. Overall, depilatory creams can be a convenient and accessible option for individuals with PCOS looking to manage unwanted hair growth and achieve hair harmony.

Laser Hair Removal:

Laser hair removal is a popular method for reducing unwanted hair growth. During the procedure, a laser device emits concentrated light energy that targets the pigment (color) in the hair follicles. The heat from the laser damages the follicles, inhibiting their ability to grow new hair. Laser hair removal is effective for treating large areas of the body, such as the face, chest, back, and legs. Multiple sessions are usually required to achieve significant hair reduction, as the treatment works best on actively growing hair. While laser hair removal can provide long-term hair reduction, maintenance sessions may be necessary to sustain results. It's important to consult with a qualified dermatologist or license practitioner to determine if laser hair removal is suitable for your individual needs and skin type.

Advantages:	Disadvantages:
Effective for large areas of the body.	Multiple sessions required for optimal results
Long-lasting results	Can be expensive.
Minimal discomfort during treatment	Not effective for light-colored or fine hair.
Suitable for various skin types	Temporary skin irritation may occur.
Quick treatment sessions.	Risk of hyperpigmentation or burns if not performed correctly

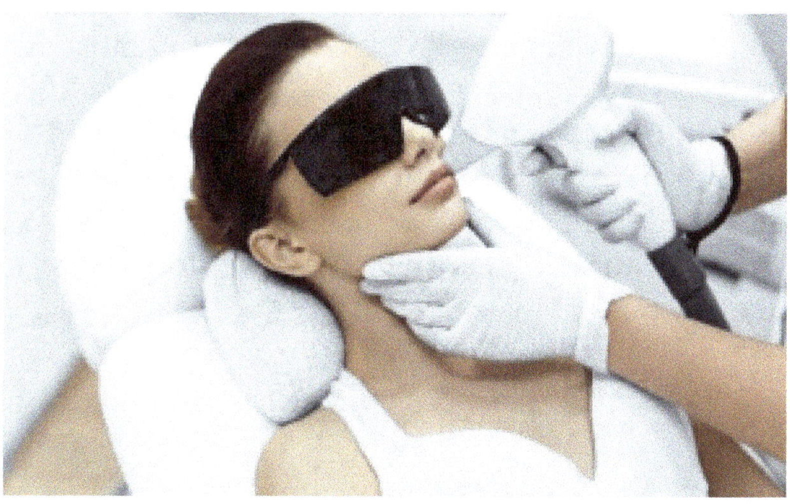

IPL (Intense Pulsed Light) Therapy

IPL therapy is a popular choice for individuals with PCOS seeking to manage unwanted hair growth. Unlike laser hair removal, which uses a single wavelength of light to target hair follicles, IPL emits multiple wavelengths in quick pulses. This broad spectrum of light penetrates the skin and is absorbed by the melanin (pigment) in the hair follicles, generating heat and damaging the follicles to inhibit future hair growth.

The key difference between laser and IPL lies in their light sources and the range of wavelengths used. While laser devices produce a concentrated beam of light at a specific wavelength, IPL devices emit a broader spectrum of light across multiple wavelengths. As a result, IPL treatments may be less precise and effective for individuals with lighter hair or darker skin tones compared to laser hair removal. However, IPL therapy offers advantages such as faster treatment times, larger treatment areas, and generally lower cost per session.

Electrolysis:

Electrolysis is another hair removal technique that can be beneficial for individuals

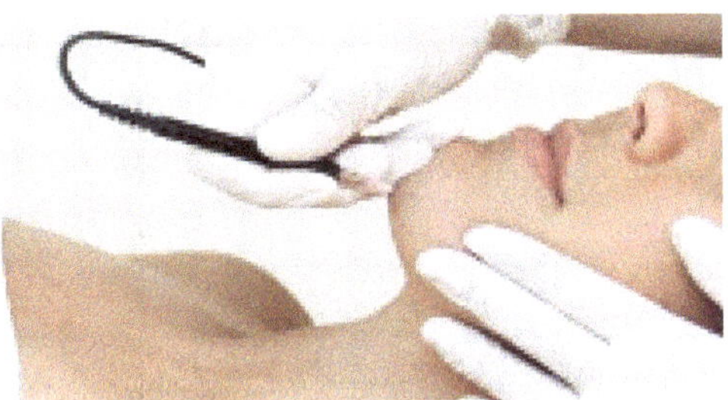

with PCOS. Unlike laser hair removal, which targets hair follicles with light energy, electrolysis uses a small electric current to destroy the hair follicles directly. During the procedure, a fine needle is inserted into each hair follicle, and electrical energy is delivered to destroy the follicle's ability to produce new hair. Electrolysis is effective for treating individual hairs or small areas of the body, making it suitable for areas with sparse or coarse hair growth, such as the chin or upper lip. Since electrolysis targets each hair follicle individually, it can be time-consuming and may require multiple sessions to achieve desired results. However, electrolysis is considered a permanent hair removal solution, making it a popular choice for individuals seeking long-lasting hair reduction. As with laser hair removal, it's essential to consult with a qualified electrologist to determine the appropriate treatment plan and ensure safety and efficacy.

Advantages	Disadvantages
Permanent hair removal solution.	Time-consuming process.
Suitable for all hair types and colors.	Can be uncomfortable or painful.
Precision targeting of individual hairs.	May require multiple sessions for optimal results.
Can be used on small areas.	Potential for skin irritation or redness.
Minimal risk of skin damage.	Higher cost compared to other hair removal methods.

CHAPTER 5:

MAINTENANCE OF HAIR & PCOS HOLLISTICAL

1. Dietary Changes
2. Food that can worsen PCOS symptoms
3. Glycemic Index
   - Low-GI Diet
   - High-GI Diet
4. Nutritional Supplements for PCOS and Hair
5. Physical Activity
6. Importance of Exercise
7. Types of Exercise
   - Aerobic Exercise
   - Resistance Training
   - Meditation
   - Breathing Exercise
   - Yoga and Pilates
8. Exercise Routine Recommendations
9. Incorporating Enjoyable Activities to Maintain Consistency

Holistic approaches look at the whole person, considering their body, mind, and lifestyle to promote overall health and well-being. When it comes to managing PCOS and hair health, holistic approaches aim to address the root causes of hormonal imbalances and support the body's natural healing processes. One important aspect of holistic care involves making dietary changes to support hormonal balance and promote healthy hair growth.

DIETARY CHANGES

Dietary changes mean making adjustments to the foods you eat every day. This can include choosing healthier options like fruits, vegetables, and whole grains, and avoiding or reducing less healthy foods like sugary snacks and processed foods. These changes can help improve your overall health and manage conditions like PCOS.

Whole Foods:

Whole foods are minimally processed and rich in nutrients, providing essential vitamins, minerals, and antioxidants. They support overall health and hormonal balance. Examples of whole foods include:

Fruits: • Apples, berries, oranges	
Vegetables: • Spinach, broccoli, carrots	
Whole Grains: • Quinoa, brown rice, oats	
Lean Proteins: • Chicken breast, fish, tofu	
Healthy Fats: • Avocado, nuts, seeds	

Balanced Carbohydrates:

Complex carbohydrates with a low glycemic index release sugar slowly into the bloodstream, preventing insulin spikes and supporting hormonal balance.

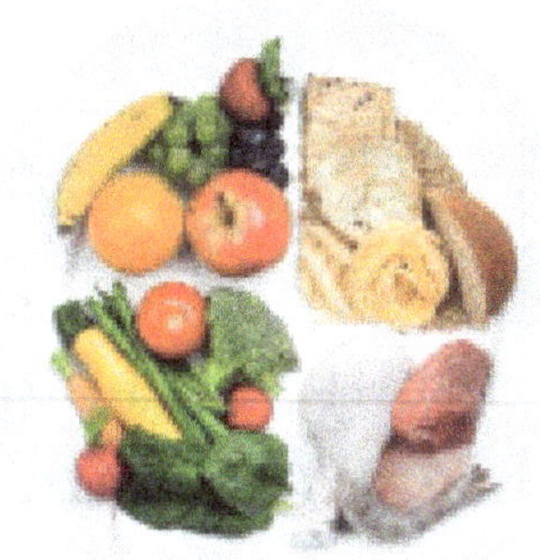

Examples of balanced carbohydrates include:

Whole Grains: - Whole wheat bread, barley, bulgur
Legumes: - Chickpeas, lentils, black beans

> **Non-Starchy Vegetables:** - Leafy greens, bell peppers, zucchini

Healthy Proteins:

Lean proteins are essential for hormone synthesis and support healthy hair growth. Examples of healthy proteins include:

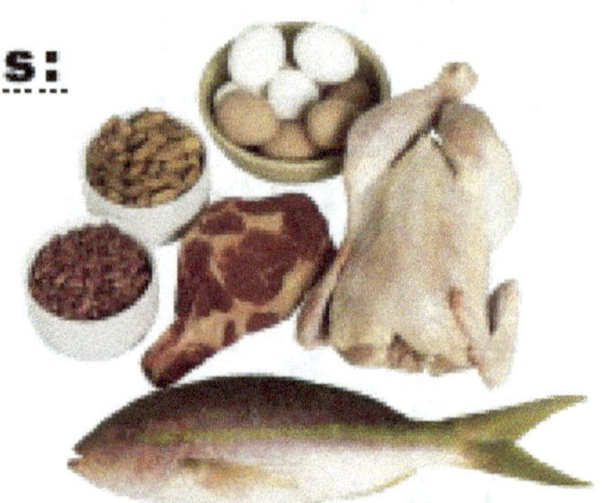

> **Poultry:** - Chicken Breast, Turkey, Lean Cuts of Beef
>
> **Fish:** - Salmon, Tuna, Trout
>
> **Plant-Based Proteins:** - Tofu, Tempeh, Edamame

Good Fats:

Healthy fats like omega-3 fatty acids reduce inflammation and support hormonal balance.

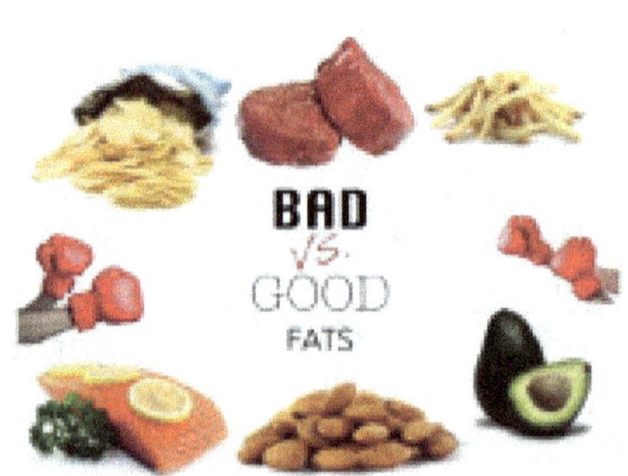

Examples of good fats include:

Nuts: - Almonds, Walnuts, Pistachios
Seeds: - Flaxseeds, Chia Seeds, Hemp Seeds
Avocado, Nuts, Olive Oil

Avoid Processed Foods and Sugars:

Processed foods and sugary snacks can cause insulin spikes, worsen insulin resistance, and disrupt hormonal balance. Examples of foods to avoid or limit include:

Fast Food: Burgers, Fries, Pizza
Sugary Snacks: Candy, Cookies, Pastries
Refined Carbohydrates: White Bread, Sugary Cereals, Pastries
Sugary Beverages: Soda, Energy Drinks, Sweetened Teas

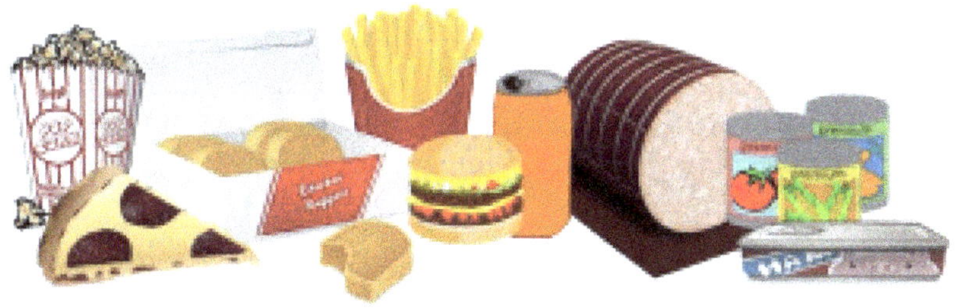

Watch Portions:

Monitoring portion sizes helps prevent overeating, weight gain, and exacerbation of PCOS symptoms. Examples of appropriate portion sizes:

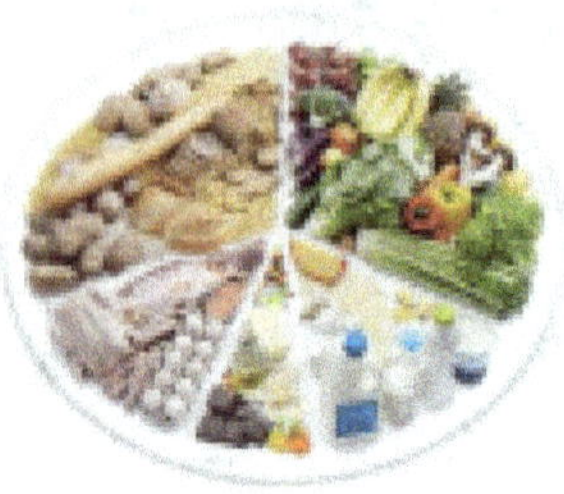

Protein: *A serving of chicken is about the size of your palm.*
Carbohydrates: *A serving of cooked grains is about half a cup.*
Fats: *A serving of nuts is about a small handful.*

Hydration:

Drinking plenty of water throughout the day supports hydration and overall health. Examples of hydrating beverages include:

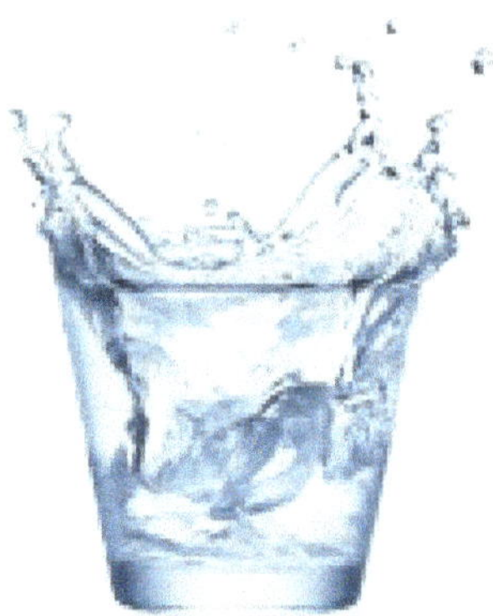

Water
Herbal Teas: *Chamomile tea, peppermint tea*
Infused Water: *Cucumber mint water, lemon ginger water*

FOODS THAT CAN WORSEN PCOS SYMPTOMS AND IMPACT HAIR HEALTH

1. Highly Processed Foods:
Foods like fast food, chips, sugary cereals, and microwave meals often contain unhealthy fats, sugars, and additives that can disrupt hormones and contribute to inflammation.

2. Sugary Treats:
Limit sugary snacks, desserts, and sweetened beverages, as they can cause blood sugar spikes and worsen insulin resistance.

3. Trans Fats:
Avoid foods containing Trans fats, such as margarine, fried foods, and commercially baked goods, as they can increase inflammation and interfere with hormone regulation.

GLYCEMIC INDEX (GI)

The GI is a ranking system that measures how quickly a carbohydrate-containing food raises your blood sugar levels. Foods with a low GI release sugar gradually, promoting stable blood sugar and insulin levels. On the other hand, high-GI foods cause spikes in blood sugar, leading to insulin surges and potential health issues.

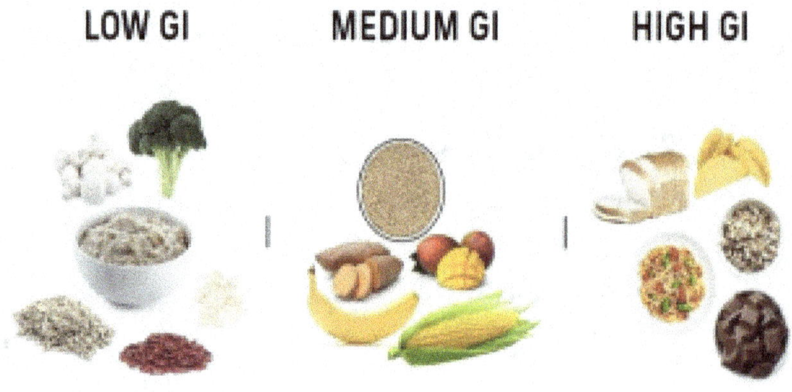

LOW-GI DIET FOR PCOS:

Many women with PCOS experience insulin resistance, meaning their bodies don't use insulin effectively. This can lead to high blood sugar

and weight gain. A low-GI diet helps manage
PCOS by:

1. Blood Sugar Control:

PCOS often involves insulin resistance,
which makes it harder for your body to use
insulin effectively. A low-GI diet can help
regulate blood sugar and improve insulin
sensitivity, potentially reducing your risk
of type 2 diabetes.

2. Weight Management:

Stable blood sugar levels can lead to better
appetite control and reduced cravings,
contributing to weight management, a
crucial aspect of PCOS management.

3. Improved Hormonal Balance:

Studies suggest that a low-GI diet may
help regulate hormone levels, potentially
reducing androgen levels associated with
PCOS symptoms like acne and excess hair
growth.

4. Enhanced Hair Health:

Stable blood sugar and reduced inflammation from a low-GI diet may contribute to improved hair growth and reduced hair loss, common concerns for many with PCOS.

TIPS FOR INCORPORATING LOW-GI FOODS:

1. Focus on Whole Foods:

Choose unprocessed grains like whole-wheat bread, brown rice, quinoa, and oats over refined options like white bread and pastries.

2. Load Up on Veggies:

Non-starchy vegetables like leafy greens, broccoli, and cauliflower are low-GI and packed with nutrients.

3. Go Lean with Protein:

Opt for lean protein sources like fish, chicken, beans, and lentils to balance your meals.

4. <u>Choose Healthy Fats:</u>

Include healthy fats like avocado, nuts, and olive oil in moderation to promote satiety and nutrient absorption.

5. <u>Limit Sugary Drinks:</u>

Replace sugary drinks with water, unsweetened tea, or coffee.

6. <u>Read Food Labels:</u>

Pay attention to the GI value listed on food labels to make informed choices.

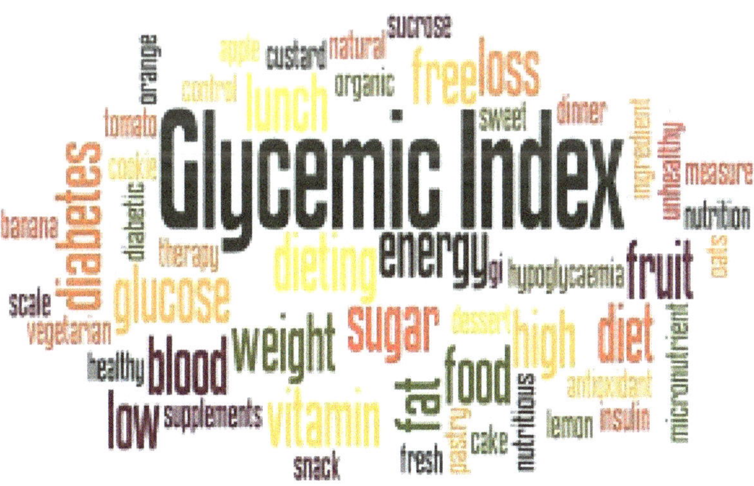

SAMPLE LOW-GI MEAL IDEAS:

BREAKFAST:

Chia Pudding: Mix chia seeds with almond milk, yogurt, or coconut milk, topped with berries, nuts, and a sprinkle of cinnamon.

Avocado Toast with Scrambled Eggs: Whole-wheat toast topped with mashed avocado, scrambled eggs, and chopped tomatoes.

Smoothie Bowl: Blend together spinach, banana, frozen berries, almond milk, and protein powder for a nutritious and filling start.

LUNCH:

Black Bean Burgers: Homemade black bean burgers on whole-wheat buns with lettuce, tomato, and a low-sugar sauce.

Tuna Salad Sandwich: Whole-wheat bread with tuna salad made with Greek yogurt, chopped celery, and Dijon mustard.

Lentil Soup with Whole-Grain Roll: Hearty lentil soup with chopped vegetables and a side of a whole-grain roll.

DINNER:

Salmon with Roasted Vegetables: Baked salmon with roasted Brussels sprouts, sweet potatoes, and onions.

Chicken Stir-fry with Brown Rice: Stir-fry chicken with mixed vegetables and brown rice, seasoned with low-sodium soy sauce and ginger.

Tofu Scramble with Whole-Wheat Tortillas: Scrambled tofu with bell peppers, onions, and spices wrapped in whole-wheat tortillas.

SNACKS:

Apple Slices with Almond Butter: A classic low-GI snack for satisfying hunger and providing healthy fats.

Hard-boiled Eggs: A good source of protein and healthy fats, perfect for on-the-go snacking.

Carrot Sticks with Hummus: A delicious and nutritious combination of fiber and protein.

Edamame: A complete protein source with a low GI value and satisfying texture.

While a low-glycemic index (GI) diet is generally recommended for managing PCOS due to its benefits in regulating blood sugar and insulin resistance, understanding the potential effects of a high-glycemic index diet can also be informative. However, it's important to remember that a high-GI diet is generally not recommended for individuals with PCOS due to its potential to worsen symptoms.

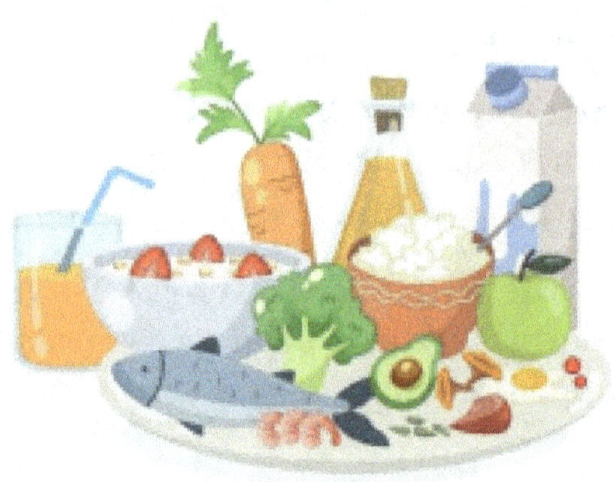

HIGH-GLYCEMIC INDEX DIET

A high-glycemic index (GI) diet consists of foods that cause rapid spikes in blood sugar levels. These foods are typically processed, refined carbohydrates, sugary drinks, and white bread. While they may provide quick energy, the associated blood sugar fluctuations can have negative consequences for overall health and can worsen PCOS symptoms.

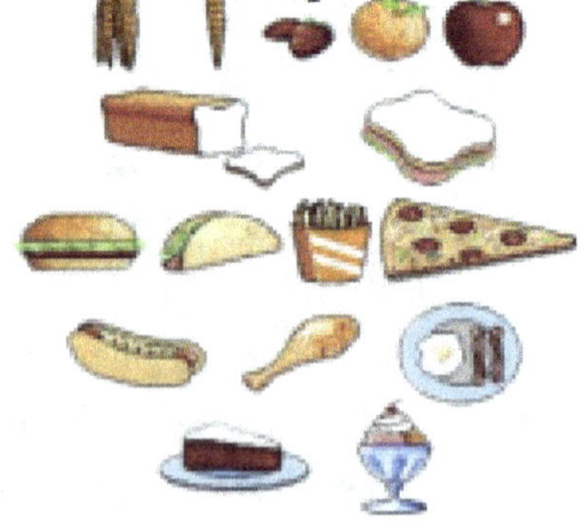

POTENTIAL DRAWBACKS OF A HIGH-GI DIET FOR PCOS:

Exacerbated insulin resistance:

The rapid rise in blood sugar caused by high-GI foods can further worsen insulin resistance, a key characteristic of PCOS. This can lead to increased weight gain, difficulty managing blood sugar levels, and an increased risk of developing type 2 diabetes.

Insulin resistance in PCOS

Hormonal imbalances: The fluctuations in blood sugar and insulin levels associated with high-GI foods can disrupt hormonal balance, potentially worsening symptoms like irregular periods, acne, and excess hair growth.

Hormonal imbalances in PCOS

Increased inflammation: Chronic inflammation is linked to PCOS, and high-GI diets can contribute to inflammation in the body, potentially worsening PCOS symptoms and increasing the risk of other health problems.

Weight gain:

High-GI foods are often calorie-dense and less satiating, leading to increased calorie intake and potential weight gain, which can worsen PCOS symptoms and overall health.

ALTERNATIVES TO A HIGH-GI DIET:

Low-glycemic index diet:

As mentioned earlier, a low-GI diet focuses on whole, unprocessed foods that release glucose slowly and steadily, helping manage blood sugar and insulin levels, potentially improving PCOS symptoms.

Mediterranean diet:

This heart-healthy diet emphasizes fruits, vegetables, whole grains, healthy fats, and lean protein, offering a balanced approach to nutrition that can benefit individuals with PCOS.

Dash diet:

This diet focuses on fruits, vegetables, whole grains, and low-fat dairy, promoting healthy blood pressure and potentially benefiting individuals with PCOS.

NUTRITIONAL SUPPLEMENTS FOR PCOS AND HAIR

Nutritional supplements are vitamins, minerals, or other substances that people take to add to their diet and support their health. They come in different forms like pills, capsules, or powders and can help fill in any nutritional gaps in our diet. Here are some key supplements that can benefit individuals with PCOS and improve hair health:

Omega-3 Fatty Acids:

Omega-3 fatty acids are healthy fats found in foods like fish, flaxseeds, and walnuts. These fats are important for overall health and can help reduce inflammation in the body, which is beneficial for individuals with PCOS. In terms of hair health, omega-3 fatty acids support a healthy scalp and hair follicles, promoting stronger and shinier hair. Including sources of omega-3s in your diet or taking supplements can help improve hair quality and manage PCOS symptoms.

Biotin:

Biotin, also known as vitamin B7, is a water-soluble vitamin that plays a crucial role in maintaining healthy hair, skin, and nails. Biotin supplements are often recommended for individuals experiencing hair thinning or hair loss, including those with PCOS. Biotin helps strengthen hair strands and promotes hair growth, resulting in thicker and fuller hair. While biotin deficiency is rare, supplementing with biotin may support hair health, particularly in individuals with PCOS who may experience hair-related concerns.

Zinc:

Zinc is an essential mineral that is involved in various physiological processes in the body, including immune function, wound healing, and DNA synthesis. Zinc also plays a role in maintaining healthy hair and may be beneficial for individuals with PCOS experiencing hair issues. Zinc deficiency has been associated with hair loss and thinning hair, so ensuring an adequate intake of zinc through diet or supplementation can support hair growth and thickness. Additionally, zinc helps regulate hormone levels in the body, which may be beneficial for individuals with PCOS who experience hormonal imbalances affecting their hair.

Incorporating these nutritional supplements into your daily routine, along with a balanced diet and lifestyle, can contribute to improved hair health and overall well-being, particularly for individuals with PCOS. However, it's important to consult with a healthcare professional before starting any new supplements to ensure they are appropriate for your individual needs and health status.

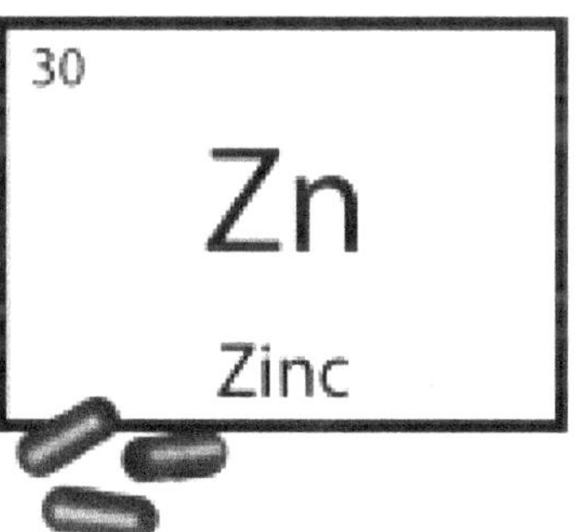

PHYSICAL ACTIVITY:

Physical activity refers to any movement that uses your muscles and burns calories. It can be anything from walking and swimming to dancing or playing sports. In PCOS, physical activity is really important for your health, including your hair. When you're active, it helps your body use insulin better, which can be tricky with PCOS. This means it can help keep your blood sugar levels stable and reduce the risk of problems like diabetes. Plus, exercise helps to lower stress, which is good because stress can make PCOS symptoms worse. When you're less stressed, your body can work better, including your hair follicles, which can lead to healthier hair. So, moving your body regularly can not only make you feel better overall but also improve the health of your hair.

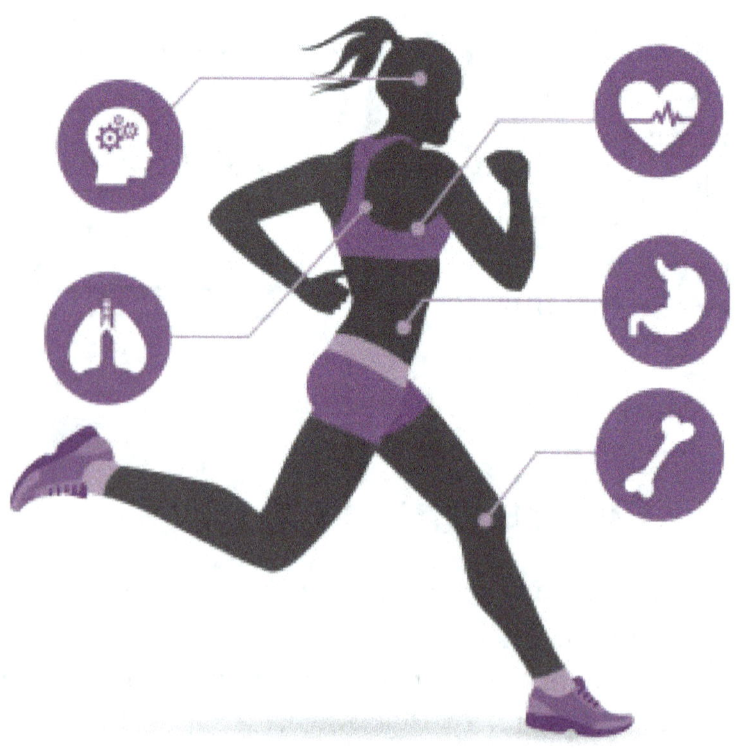

IMPORTANCE OF EXERCISE

Regulation of Insulin Levels:

Exercise plays a crucial role in regulating insulin levels in the body, especially for individuals with PCOS who may experience insulin resistance. Insulin resistance occurs when cells in the body don't respond effectively to insulin, leading to high blood sugar levels. Regular physical activity helps improve insulin sensitivity, allowing cells to better absorb glucose from the bloodstream and thereby reducing the risk of high blood sugar levels and diabetes. By incorporating exercise into their routine, individuals with PCOS can better manage their insulin levels and promote overall metabolic health.

Reduction of Stress:

Exercise is also known to be a natural stress reliever. For individuals with PCOS, managing stress levels is important as stress can exacerbate hormonal imbalances and worsen symptoms such as irregular periods, acne, and hair issues. Engaging in physical activity triggers the release of endorphins, which are chemicals in the brain that help reduce stress and improve mood. Regular exercise can help individuals with PCOS better cope with stressors in their daily lives, leading to improved emotional well-being and hormonal balance.

Improvement in Overall Health and Well-being:

Beyond its effects on insulin regulation and stress reduction, exercise offers numerous benefits for overall health and well-being. Regular physical activity helps strengthen the cardiovascular system, improve muscle tone and flexibility, and enhance immune function. It also promotes weight management by burning calories and increasing metabolism, which is particularly beneficial for individuals with PCOS who may struggle with weight gain. Additionally, exercise can improve sleep quality, boost energy levels, and increase self-esteem and confidence. By incorporating regular exercise into their lifestyle, individuals with PCOS can improve their overall health and enhance their quality of life.

<u>TYPES OF EXERCISE</u>

<u>Aerobic Exercises</u>

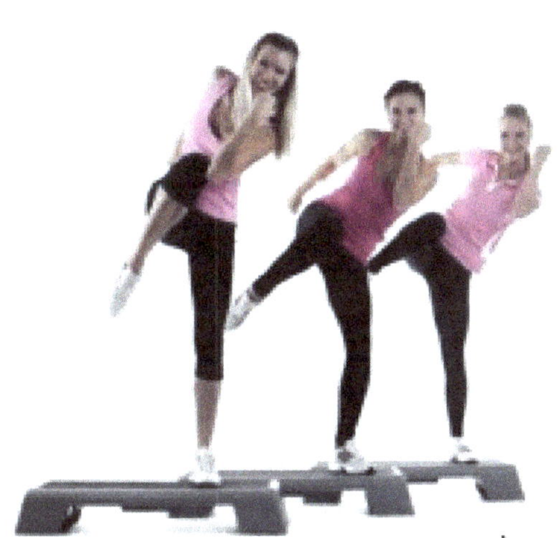

Aerobic exercises, such as walking, jogging, and swimming, can be really helpful for women with PCOS who are looking to improve their hair health and overall well-being. These exercises get your heart pumping and your blood flowing, which can help improve circulation throughout your body, including your scalp. This increased blood flow delivers more oxygen and nutrients to your hair follicles, promoting hair growth and strengthening your hair. Additionally, aerobic exercises can help reduce levels of certain hormones associated with PCOS, like insulin and androgens, which may contribute to hair issues such as excess hair growth or hair thinning. Plus, these exercises are great for managing weight, improving mood, and reducing stress, all of which can indirectly support healthier hair. So, incorporating regular aerobic exercises into your routine can be a positive step towards achieving hair harmony and overall wellness with PCOS.

List of Aerobic Exercises

Walking	Jumping Rope
Jogging/Running	Aerobic Classes (e.g Zumba)
Swimming	Hiking
Cycling	Elliptical Machine
Dancing	Rowing

Resistance Training:

Resistance training, which includes exercises like weightlifting and bodyweight exercises, can be beneficial for individuals with PCOS to promote hair harmony. When we do resistance training, our muscles work against a force, like lifting weights or doing push-ups. This type of exercise helps to increase muscle strength and mass, improve metabolism, and regulate insulin levels. In PCOS, resistance training can help manage hormonal imbalances by increasing insulin sensitivity, which may reduce the production of androgens, the male hormones that can contribute to hair issues like hirsutism and hair loss.

Additionally, resistance training can support overall health and well-being by reducing stress, promoting better sleep, and boosting confidence. Including resistance training as part of a comprehensive exercise routine can contribute to better hair health and harmony.

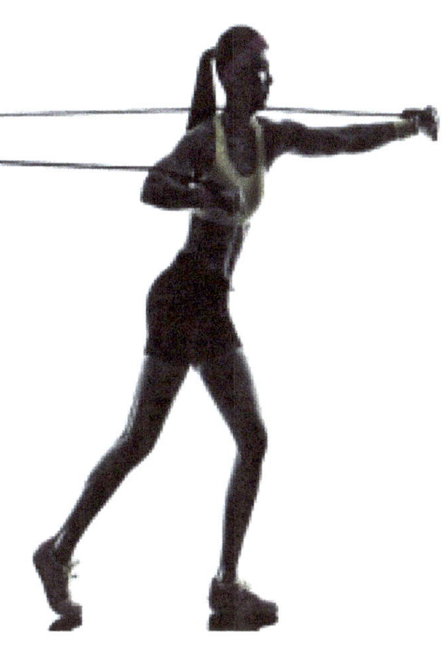

List of Resistance Exercises:

Squats	Leg Press
Lunges	Leg Curl
Deadlifts	Leg Extension
Bench Press	Calf Raises
Shoulder Press	Planks
Bent-over Rows	Russian Twists
Pull-ups/Chin-ups	Bicycle Crunches
Push-ups	Superman
Tricep Dips	Glute Bridge
Bicep Curls	Dumbbell Flyes

<u>MEDITATION</u>

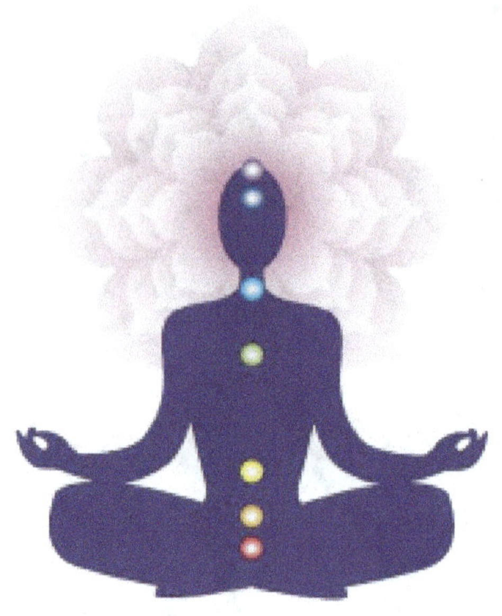

Meditation is a practice that involves training the mind to focus and redirect thoughts. It's often used to promote relaxation, reduce stress, and enhance overall well-being. In the context of PCOS and hair harmony, meditation can be particularly beneficial

When someone has PCOS, hormonal imbalances and associated symptoms like hirsutism (excess hair growth) or hair loss can cause stress and anxiety. Meditation can help manage these emotions by calming the mind and reducing stress levels. This, in turn, may positively impact hormone levels and potentially improve hair health.

Additionally, stress is known to contribute to hormonal imbalances, which can exacerbate PCOS symptoms. By incorporating meditation into their daily routine, individuals with PCOS may experience better hormonal regulation, leading to improvements in hair growth patterns and overall health.

Moreover, meditation can enhance self-awareness and mindfulness, allowing individuals to better understand their bodies and recognize any changes or patterns in their symptoms. This self-awareness can empower individuals with PCOS to take proactive steps towards managing their condition, including adopting healthy lifestyle habits and seeking appropriate medical care.

Overall, incorporating meditation into a comprehensive approach to managing PCOS and promoting hair harmony can have numerous benefits, including stress reduction, improved hormone balance, and enhanced overall well-being.

BREATHING EXERCISES

Breathing exercises can be really helpful for managing PCOS and promoting hair harmony. When we're stressed, our bodies can release hormones like cortisol, which can disrupt our hormonal balance and affect our hair health. By practicing breathing exercises, we can reduce stress levels and help our bodies relax, which in turn can support hormonal balance and improve hair growth.

One simple breathing exercise you can try is deep belly breathing. Find a quiet, comfortable place to sit or lie down. Close your eyes and place one hand on your belly. Take a slow, deep breath in through your nose, feeling your belly rise as you fill your lungs with air. Hold your breath for a moment, then slowly exhale through your mouth, feeling your belly fall as you release the air. Repeat this process for several minutes, focusing on your breath and letting go of any tension or stress you may be holding onto.

Another helpful breathing technique is called the 4-7-8 breath. Start by exhaling completely through your mouth, making a whooshing sound as you release all the air from your lungs. Then, close your mouth and inhale quietly through your nose for a count of four seconds. Hold your breath for a count of seven seconds. Finally, exhale slowly through your mouth, making a whooshing sound, for a count of eight seconds. Repeat this cycle for several rounds, allowing yourself to relax more deeply with each breath.

By incorporating these breathing exercises into your daily routine, you can support your body's natural ability to manage stress, promote hormonal balance, and maintain healthy hair growth. Remember to be patient with yourself and practice regularly to experience the full benefits of these techniques.

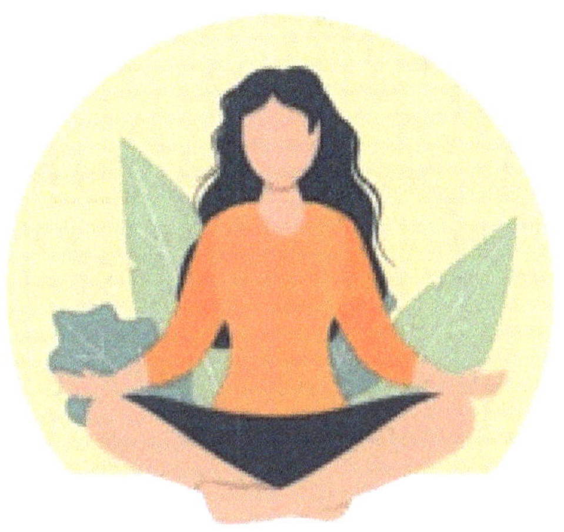

YOGA AND PILATES FOR STRESS REDUCTION AND FLEXIBILITY IN PCOS

In the journey of managing PCOS and maintaining healthy hair, finding effective stress reduction techniques is essential. Yoga and Pilates are two popular forms of exercise known for their ability to reduce stress levels and improve flexibility. In this section, we will explore how practicing yoga and Pilates can benefit individuals with PCOS by reducing stress and promoting overall well-being, including healthy hair growth.

Yoga for Stress Reduction and Flexibility:

Yoga is a holistic practice that combines physical postures (asanas), breathing techniques (pranayama), and meditation to promote relaxation and inner peace. For individuals with PCOS, who often experience elevated stress levels due to hormonal imbalances, practicing yoga can be highly beneficial. Yoga helps to reduce cortisol levels (the stress hormone) in the

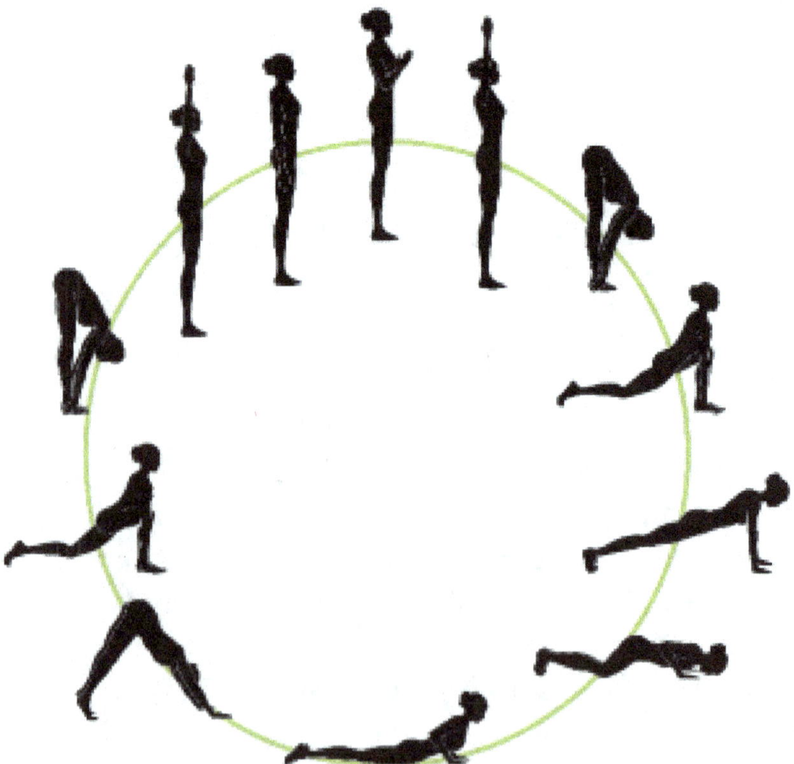

body, thereby alleviating stress and anxiety. Additionally, certain yoga poses can improve flexibility, which is important for overall physical health and may indirectly support hair health by improving circulation to the scalp.

Pilates for Stress Reduction and Flexibility:

Pilates is a low-impact exercise system that focuses on strengthening the core muscles, improving posture, and enhancing flexibility. Like yoga, Pilates can help reduce stress by promoting mindfulness and relaxation through controlled movements and breathing techniques. By strengthening the core and stabilizing the body, Pilates also helps improve overall body awareness and coordination, which can have positive effects on mental well-being. Moreover, Pilates exercises often involve stretching and lengthening the muscles, leading to improved flexibility and mobility, which can support overall physical health and potentially aid in maintaining healthy hair.

Incorporating Yoga and Pilates into Your Routine:

To experience the benefits of yoga and Pilates for stress reduction and flexibility, it's essential to incorporate regular practice into your routine. Start with beginner-friendly classes or online tutorials tailored to your fitness level and physical abilities. Set aside dedicated time each week for yoga and Pilates sessions, aiming for at least 2-3 sessions per week to reap the maximum benefits. Remember to listen to your body and modify poses as needed to avoid strain or injury.

List of Exercises for Yoga for Stress Reduction and Flexibility

Child's Pose (Balasana)	Bridge Pose (Setu Bandhasana)
Cat-Cow Stretch (Marjaryasana-Bitilasana)	Warrior I (Virabhadrasana I)
Downward-Facing Dog (Adho Mukha Svanasana)	Warrior II (Virabhadrasana II)
Forward Fold (Uttanasana)	Tree Pose (Vrksasana)
Seated Forward Bend (Paschimottanasana)	Legs-Up-the-Wall Pose (Viparita Karani)
Cobra Pose (Bhujangasana)	Corpse Pose (Savasana)

List of Exercises for Pilates for Stress Reduction and Flexibility:

Pelvic Curl	Saw
Hundred	Swan Dive Prep
Roll-Up	Swan
Single Leg Stretch	Side Leg Kick
Double Leg Stretch	Mermaid Stretch
Spine Stretch Forward	Corkscrew

EXERCISE ROUTINE RECOMMENDATIONS

Exercise is important for everyone, including those with PCOS, to help manage symptoms and promote overall health, including hair health. Here's a breakdown of exercise routine recommendations tailored for individuals with PCOS:

Frequency:

Aim for at least 150 minutes of moderate-intensity aerobic exercise per week, spread out over several days. This could mean doing activities like brisk walking, cycling, swimming, or dancing for about 30 minutes on most days of the week.

Duration:

Each exercise session should ideally last for about 30 minutes to an hour. However, if you're just starting out, you can begin with shorter sessions and gradually increase the duration as you build up your fitness level.

Intensity:

Choose exercises that get your heart rate up and make you break a sweat, but you should still be able to talk comfortably while exercising. This is known as moderate-intensity exercise. If you prefer more vigorous activities, like running or high-intensity interval training (HIIT), aim for at least 75 minutes per week.

Incorporate Strength Training:

In addition to aerobic exercise, include strength training exercises at least two days a week. This could involve using weights, resistance bands, or bodyweight exercises like squats, lunges, and push-ups. Strength training helps build muscle mass, which can improve metabolism and hormone regulation in individuals with PCOS.

Be Consistent:

Consistency is key when it comes to exercise. Aim to make physical activity a regular part of your routine, scheduling workouts at times that work best for you and sticking to your plan as much as possible.

Listen to Your Body:

Pay attention to how your body responds to exercise and adjust your routine accordingly. If you experience any discomfort or pain, modify your activities or seek guidance from a healthcare professional or fitness expert

Remember that finding an exercise routine that you enjoy and can stick to is important for long-term success. Experiment with different activities to see what you like best and what fits into your lifestyle. By staying active, you can not only improve your overall health but also support hair harmony and manage PCOS symptoms effectively.

INCORPORATING ENJOYABLE ACTIVITIES TO MAINTAIN CONSISTENCY

Incorporating enjoyable activities is essential for maintaining consistency in managing PCOS and promoting hair harmony. When dealing with PCOS, it's important to adopt healthy lifestyle habits that you enjoy and can stick with over time. This helps to maintain hormonal balance, which is crucial for managing PCOS symptoms, including those related to hair health.

Firstly, finding physical activities that you enjoy can be beneficial for managing PCOS symptoms and promoting overall well-being. Exercise helps to regulate insulin levels, improve metabolism, and reduce stress, all of which can positively impact hair health. Whether it's walking, dancing, swimming, or yoga, choose activities that you find enjoyable and incorporate them into your regular routine.

Additionally, incorporating stress-reducing activities can be beneficial for managing PCOS and supporting hair harmony. High levels of stress can exacerbate hormonal imbalances and lead to hair-related issues such as hair loss or thinning. Engaging in activities like meditation, deep breathing exercises, or spending time in nature can help to lower stress levels and promote relaxation, which can have a positive impact on hair health.

Furthermore, prioritizing self-care activities that you enjoy can contribute to maintaining consistency in managing PCOS and promoting hair harmony. This can include indulging in hobbies you love, spending time with loved ones, or pampering yourself with a relaxing bath or skincare routine. Taking time for yourself and doing activities that bring you joy can help to reduce stress levels and improve overall well-being, which can have a positive impact on hair health.

Overall, incorporating enjoyable activities into your routine is important for maintaining consistency in managing PCOS and promoting hair harmony. By finding activities that you love and incorporating them into your daily life, you can support hormonal balance, reduce stress, and improve overall well-being, which can have a positive impact on your hair health and overall quality of life

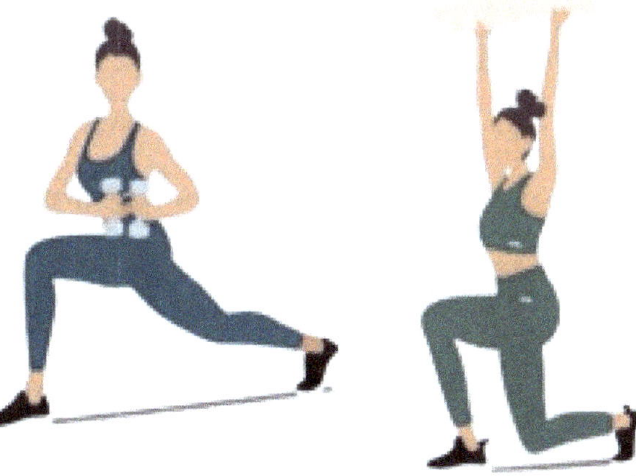

CHAPTER 6:

PCOS PSYCHOLOGICAL WELL-BEING AND HAIR HEALTH

1. Importance of Addressing Psychological Well-Being in Managing PCOS-Related Hair Concerns
2. Emotional Challenges Associated with PCOS Diagnosis
   - Diagnosis Shock and Uncertainty
   - Body Image Issues
   - Fertility Concerns
   - Social Stigma and Isolation
3. Impact of Hormonal Imbalances on Mood, Self-Esteem, And Body Image In PCOS
4. Psychological Effects of Hair Loss in PCOS
5. Psychological Effects of Hirsutism in PCOS
6. Coping Mechanisms for Managing Hair-Related Psychological Issues in PCOS
7. Strategies for Coping with Emotional Challenges and Achieving Hair Harmony
8. Role of Healthcare Providers in Addressing Psychological Concerns and Providing Emotional Support

Our mental and emotional health can have a big impact on the health of our hair, especially for those with conditions like Polycystic Ovary Syndrome (PCOS). When we talk about psychological well-being, we're referring to how we feel emotionally and mentally. It's about feeling good about ourselves, managing stress, and coping with life's ups and downs.

Now, let's look at how our mental and emotional health can affect our hair. When we're stressed or anxious, our bodies release certain hormones that can disrupt the normal cycle of hair growth. This can lead to issues like hair loss or thinning. Similarly, conditions like depression can affect our self-care routines, including how well we take care of our hair and scalp.

When it comes to PCOS, the hormonal imbalances associated with the condition can also impact hair health. For example, higher levels of androgens (male hormones) in women with PCOS can cause excess hair growth on the face, chest, or back (hirsutism), while also contributing to hair loss on the scalp.

So, there's a clear link between our emotional well-being and the health of our hair. When we're feeling good mentally and emotionally, it can positively impact the growth and appearance of our hair. On the other hand, when we're struggling with stress, anxiety, or depression, it can manifest in our hair health.

IMPORTANCE OF ADDRESSING PSYCHOLOGICAL WELL-BEING IN MANAGING PCOS-RELATED HAIR CONCERNS

Addressing psychological well-being is crucial when managing hair concerns related to PCOS, as these issues can significantly impact a person's overall quality of life. PCOS-related hair changes, such as excessive hair growth (hirsutism) or hair loss (alopecia), can have profound psychological effects, leading to feelings of embarrassment, low self-esteem, and even depression or anxiety.

Firstly, it's essential to recognize that hair concerns are not merely cosmetic issues but can deeply affect how individuals perceive themselves and interact with others. Hirsutism, for example, can cause distress and social withdrawal due to societal beauty standards and expectations. Similarly, hair loss can be emotionally challenging, particularly for women, as thick and healthy hair is often associated with femininity and attractiveness.

Furthermore, the hormonal imbalances characteristic of PCOS can exacerbate emotional distress. Fluctuating hormone levels can contribute to mood swings, irritability, and anxiety, amplifying the emotional impact of hair concerns. Additionally, the stigma surrounding PCOS and its visible symptoms may lead to feelings of isolation and shame, further affecting psychological well-being.

To address these psychological challenges effectively, a holistic approach to PCOS management is essential. This approach should include not only medical interventions to address hormonal imbalances and hair concerns but also psychological support and coping strategies. Encouraging open communication about feelings and concerns related to hair changes, providing education and reassurance, and offering counseling or therapy can all help individuals navigate the emotional aspects of PCOS-related hair concerns.

Moreover, promoting self-care practices and building self-confidence are integral parts of managing psychological well-being in PCOS. Encouraging individuals to focus on activities that bring them joy and fulfillment, practicing self-compassion, and cultivating a positive body image can help mitigate the negative impact of hair concerns on mental health.

EMOTIONAL CHALLENGES ASSOCIATED WITH PCOS DIAGNOSIS

PCOS, or Polycystic Ovary Syndrome, is a complex condition with far-reaching effects beyond physical symptoms. While irregular periods, acne, and excess hair growth are often discussed, the emotional toll of PCOS can be just as significant and shouldn't be overlooked.

Diagnosis Shock & Uncertainty:

Receiving a PCOS diagnosis can feel like a big shock. You might feel overwhelmed and confused because you weren't expecting it or because you don't fully understand what it means. Suddenly, you have this condition that you might not have even heard of before, and you're not sure what it will mean for your life. You might have lots of questions about what PCOS is, how it will affect you, and what you can do about it. It's normal to feel scared or anxious about what the future holds when you're facing something new and uncertain like this.

Body Image Issues:

Polycystic Ovary Syndrome (PCOS) can affect how you see yourself and feel about your body.

CHANGES IN APPEARANCE	PCOS can bring about physical changes that might not make you feel good about yourself. For example, you might gain weight, get acne, or have more hair than you'd like in places like your face, chest, or back.
FEELING SELF-CONSCIOUS	When these changes happen, you might start to feel self-conscious or embarrassed about how you look. You might worry about what other people think or feel uncomfortable in your own skin.
IMPACT ON CONFIDENCE	Dealing with these changes can take a toll on your confidence. You might not feel as good about yourself as you used to, and it can be hard to feel confident when you're not happy with how you look.
NEGATIVE BODY IMAGE	PCOS-related changes may lead to negative body image, where you constantly focus on perceived flaws and feel

	dissatisfied with your appearance. This negative body image can take a toll on your mental well-being and quality of life.
COMPARISON WITH OTHERS	Comparing yourself to others, especially those without PCOS or who have different body types, may exacerbate feelings of inadequacy or insecurity. Constantly measuring yourself against unrealistic standards can further damage self-esteem.
IMPACT ON INTIMATE RELATIONSHIPS	Feeling self-conscious about your body due to PCOS symptoms can impact intimate relationships and sexual confidence. Fear of rejection or judgment from partners may create barriers to intimacy and affect overall relationship satisfaction.
CLOTHING CHALLENGES	Changes in body shape and size due to PCOS-related weight gain may make it challenging to find clothes that fit comfortably and flatter your figure. Shopping for clothes can become a source of

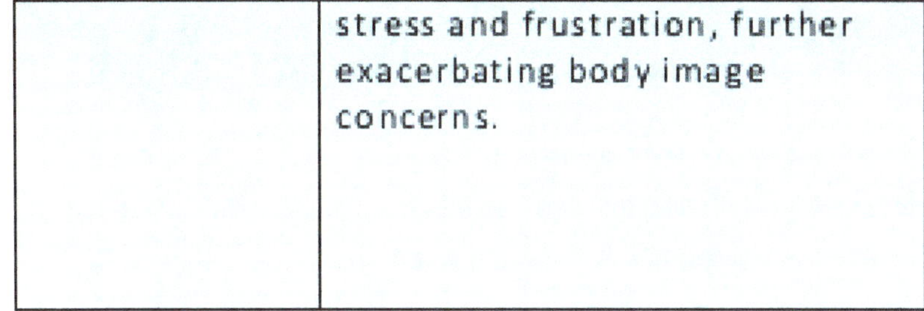

It's important to know that it's okay to struggle with how you feel about your body. PCOS can bring about a lot of changes, and it's normal to feel upset or frustrated about them. It's okay to ask for help or support if you need it. Remember that you are more than your appearance. Focus on the things you like about yourself and the things you're good at. Surround yourself with people who support you and make you feel good about yourself.

Fertility Concerns:

Fertility concerns can be a significant worry for women with PCOS. PCOS can make it harder to get pregnant because it can affect ovulation, which is when an egg is released from the ovaries. Without ovulation, it's much more challenging to conceive a baby. Many women with PCOS worry about whether they'll be able to have children at all, and this uncertainty can lead to feelings of sadness, frustration, or even grief. It's tough to face the possibility that starting a family might not happen as easily as you hoped, and it's okay to feel upset about it.

Dealing with fertility concerns means facing difficult emotions and making tough decisions. Some women with PCOS may need medical help to get pregnant, like fertility treatments or medications to help them ovulate. Others might explore alternative options, like adoption or surrogacy. No matter what path you choose, it's essential to have support from loved ones and healthcare professionals who understand what you're going through. You're not alone in your fertility journey, and there are ways to navigate these challenges with hope and resilience.

Social Stigma & Isolation:

PCOS is a condition that many people still don't know much about, and because of this, there can be a lot of misunderstandings and unfair judgments. People might not understand how PCOS affects you, and they might make assumptions or say things that hurt your feelings. This can make you feel like you're being judged or ashamed of having PCOS. It's tough when others don't get what you're going through, and it can make you feel really lonely, like you're the only one dealing with this. But it's essential to remember that you're not alone, and there are people who understand and can support you through it. It's okay to reach out for help and to talk about how you're feeling.

IMPACT OF HORMONAL IMBALANCES ON MOOD, SELF-ESTEEM, AND BODY IMAGE IN PCOS

When you have Polycystic Ovary Syndrome (PCOS), hormonal imbalances can affect more than just your physical health. They can also have a big impact on your emotions and how you see yourself. Here's how:

Mood Swings:

Hormonal fluctuations in PCOS can cause mood swings, which means your emotions might go up and down unpredictably. One moment, you might feel happy and energetic, and the next, you could feel sad or irritable for no apparent reason. This can make it tough to regulate your emotions

and can affect your overall mood and well-being.

Anxiety and Depression:

Many people with PCOS struggle with feelings of anxiety or depression. Hormonal imbalances can contribute to these mental health issues, making you feel constantly worried, tense, or overwhelmed. Depression can also make you feel sad, hopeless, or unmotivated, impacting your ability to enjoy life and engage in daily activities.

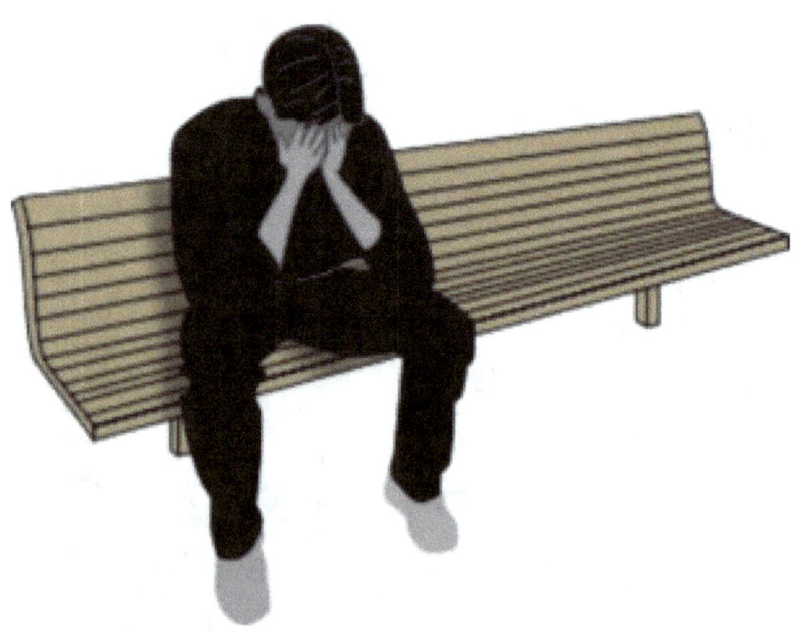

Self-Esteem:

PCOS symptoms like acne, excessive hair growth, or hair loss can affect how you feel about yourself. You might feel self-conscious or embarrassed about these visible signs of PCOS, leading to a decrease in self-esteem. Feeling uncomfortable in your own skin can impact your confidence and make it harder to feel good about yourself.

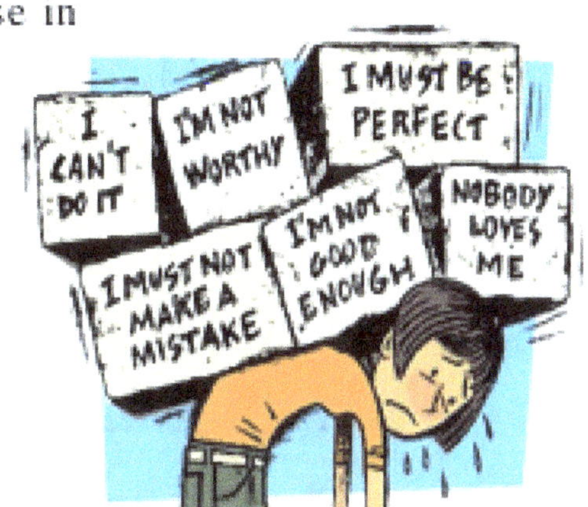

Body Image:

Weight gain is a common symptom of PCOS, and it can be challenging to manage. Hormonal imbalances can make it harder to lose weight, even with diet and exercise. This can lead to feelings of frustration, dissatisfaction with your body, and negative body image. You might compare

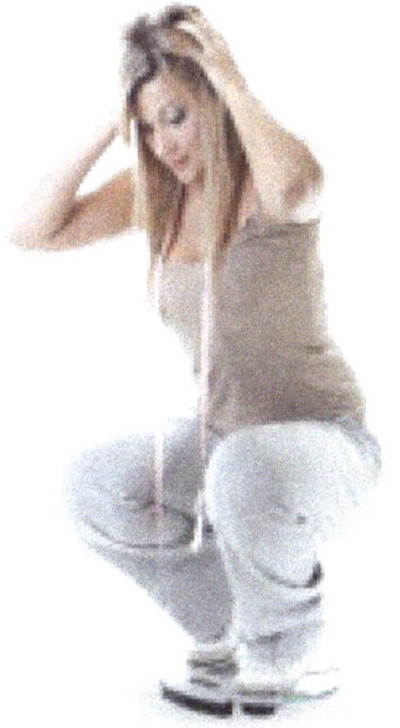

yourself to others or feel pressure to meet certain beauty standards, further affecting how you perceive your body.

Dealing with the emotional impact of PCOS can be tough, but it's essential to remember that you're not alone. Remember to be kind to yourself and prioritize self-care as you navigate the emotional ups and downs of living with PCOS.

PSYCHOLOGICAL EFFECTS OF HAIR LOSS IN PCOS

Hair loss is a common concern for individuals with Polycystic Ovary Syndrome (PCOS), and it can have significant psychological effects on mental well-being. When experiencing hair loss, individuals may feel a range of emotions, including sadness, frustration, and anxiety. This emotional response is understandable as hair loss can affect self-esteem and body image.

For many people, hair is an important part of their identity and losing it can feel like losing a part of themselves. This can lead to feelings of insecurity and self-consciousness, especially if hair loss is noticeable or occurs in highly visible areas such as the scalp or face. Additionally, societal beauty standards often place a strong emphasis on having a full head of hair, which can further exacerbate feelings of inadequacy or unattractiveness.

The psychological effects of hair loss in PCOS can also impact social interactions and relationships. Individuals may avoid social situations or feel uncomfortable being seen in public, fearing judgment or negative reactions from others. This can lead to isolation and withdrawal from social activities, which can further contribute to feelings of loneliness and depression

PSYCHOLOGICAL EFFECTS OF HIRSUTISM IN PCOS

Hirsutism is a condition where excessive hair growth occurs in areas of the body where men typically grow hair, such as the face, chest, or back. When hirsutism is associated with Polycystic Ovary Syndrome (PCOS), it can have significant psychological effects on individuals.

PCOS is a hormonal disorder that affects people who have ovaries. It can cause various symptoms, including irregular periods, weight gain, and hormonal imbalances. One common symptom of PCOS is hirsutism, which can be distressing for many individuals.

Imagine waking up one day to find hair growing on your face or chest where you never had it before. This sudden change in appearance can be shocking and embarrassing. It may make you feel self-conscious and insecure about your looks, affecting your confidence and self-esteem.

People with PCOS-related hirsutism often experience negative emotions like shame, embarrassment, or frustration. They may worry about how others perceive them and feel pressured to hide or cover up their excess hair, leading to feelings of isolation and social withdrawal.

The psychological impact of hirsutism in PCOS can also extend to relationships and daily life. Individuals may avoid social gatherings or intimate relationships due to fear of judgment or rejection. They may struggle with feelings of depression or anxiety, affecting their overall well-being and quality of life.

COPING MECHANISMS FOR MANAGING HAIR-RELATED PSYCHOLOGICAL ISSUES IN PCOS

When individuals with Polycystic Ovary Syndrome (PCOS) experience hair-related concerns like hair loss or hirsutism (excessive hair growth), it can have a significant impact on their psychological well-being. Coping mechanisms are strategies or techniques that people use to manage and alleviate the emotional distress associated with these hair-related issues. Here are some common coping mechanisms employed by individuals with PCOS

Seeking Support:

Many individuals find comfort and validation by talking about their hair-related concerns with trusted friends, family members, or support groups. Sharing experiences and feelings with others who understand can help reduce feelings of isolation and provide emotional support.

Educating Themselves:

Learning more about PCOS and its effects on hair growth patterns can empower individuals to better understand their condition and make informed decisions about treatment options. Knowledge about the underlying causes of hair loss or hirsutism can also reduce anxiety and uncertainty.

Developing Self-Care Practices:

Engaging in self-care activities such as practicing mindfulness, meditation, or relaxation techniques can help reduce stress and promote emotional well-being. Taking time for activities that bring joy and relaxation, such as hobbies or leisure activities, can also be beneficial.

Exploring Treatment Options:

Seeking medical or dermatological treatment for hair-related concerns can provide tangible solutions and improve self-esteem. Treatment options may include medications, topical treatments, laser therapy, or cosmetic procedures to manage hair loss or hirsutism.

Embracing Body Positivity:

Adopting a body-positive mindset and practicing self-acceptance can help individuals with PCOS feel more confident and comfortable in their own skin, regardless of their hair-related issues. Surrounding oneself with positive affirmations and supportive social circles can reinforce a healthy body image.

Setting Realistic Expectations:

Understanding that managing hair-related concerns in PCOS may take time and patience can help individuals set realistic expectations for their progress. Celebrating small victories and milestones along the way can boost morale and motivation.

Seeking Professional Help:

Consulting with healthcare professionals such as endocrinologists, dermatologists, or mental health therapists can provide personalized guidance and support tailored to individual needs. Therapeutic interventions such as cognitive-behavioral therapy (CBT) or acceptance and commitment therapy (ACT) can help individuals develop effective coping strategies and improve resilience in dealing with hair-related psychological issues.

By implementing these coping mechanisms, individuals with PCOS can better manage the emotional challenges associated with hair-related concerns and cultivate a sense of empowerment and resilience in their journey toward hair harmony and psychological well-being.

<u>STRATEGIES FOR COPING WITH EMOTIONAL CHALLENGES AND ACHIEVING HAIR HARMONY</u>

When you're dealing with PCOS, it's not just about managing physical symptoms; it's also essential to take care of your mental and emotional health. Psychological well-being refers to how you feel emotionally and mentally, and it plays a crucial role in overall wellness. Here, we'll discuss some helpful strategies for navigating the emotional challenges associated with PCOS while promoting harmony and confidence in your hair.

<u>Counseling and Therapy:</u>

Counseling or therapy can be incredibly beneficial for individuals with PCOS who are struggling with feelings of anxiety, depression, or low self-esteem. A trained therapist can provide a safe space for you to explore your emotions, identify coping strategies, and develop skills to manage stress and improve self-esteem. Through regular sessions, you can gain valuable insights into your thoughts and feelings and learn effective ways to navigate the challenges of living with PCOS.

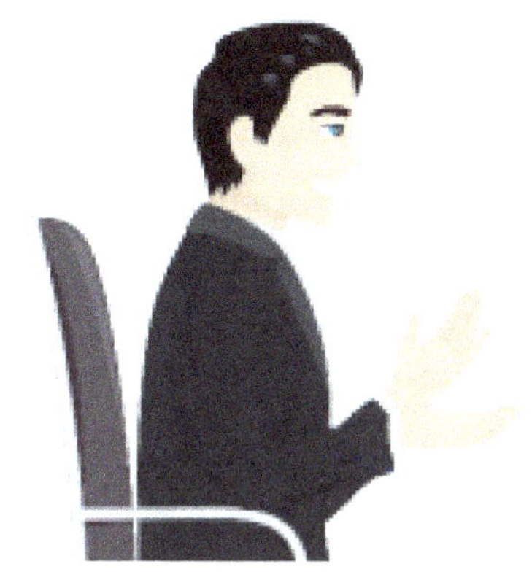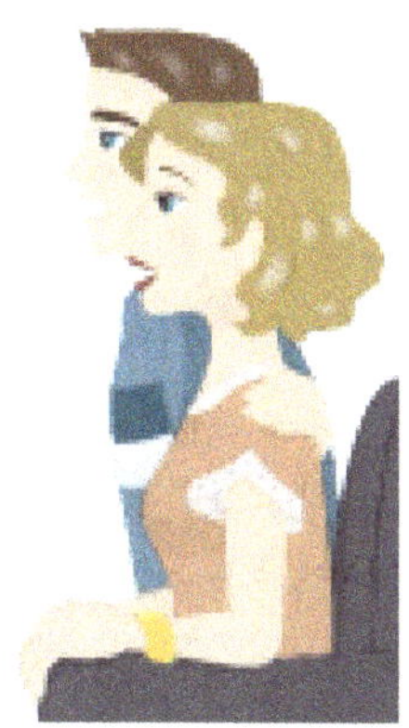

<u>Support Groups:</u>

Joining a support group for individuals with PCOS can provide invaluable emotional support and encouragement. Connecting with others who understand what you're going through can help you feel less alone and isolated. Support groups offer a platform to share experiences, exchange advice, and receive validation from peers facing similar challenges. Whether in-person or online, these communities can be a source of comfort and empowerment as you navigate your PCOS journey.

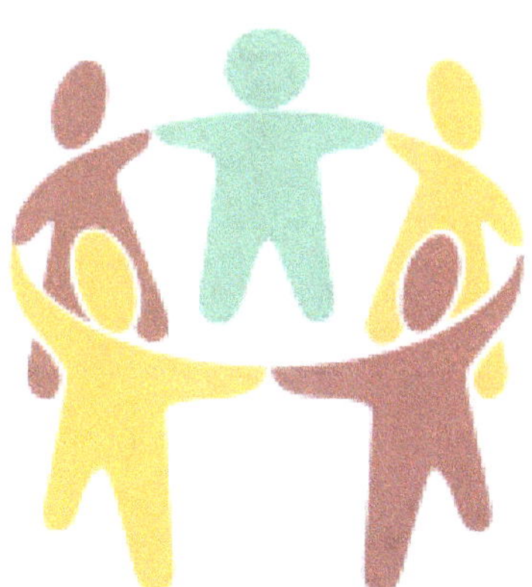

Mindfulness Techniques:

Mindfulness techniques, such as meditation, deep breathing exercises, and mindfulness-based stress reduction (MBSR) practices, can help alleviate stress and promote emotional well-being. By focusing on the present moment and cultivating awareness of your thoughts and feelings without judgment, mindfulness can help you manage anxiety, reduce rumination, and enhance self-awareness. Integrating mindfulness into your daily routine can provide a sense of calm and balance amidst the ups and downs of living with PCOS.

Incorporating these strategies into your self-care routine can help you cultivate resilience, cope with the emotional challenges of PCOS, and promote psychological well-being. By prioritizing your mental and emotional health, you can better navigate the complexities of PCOS while fostering harmony and confidence in your relationship with your hair.

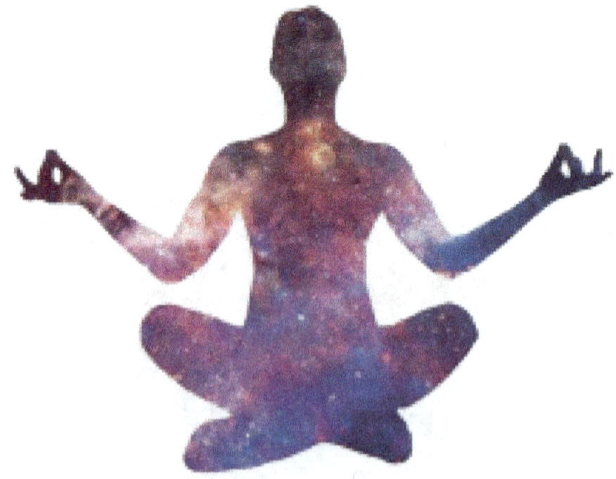

ROLE OF HEALTHCARE PROVIDERS IN ADDRESSING PSYCHOLOGICAL CONCERNS AND PROVIDING EMOTIONAL SUPPORT

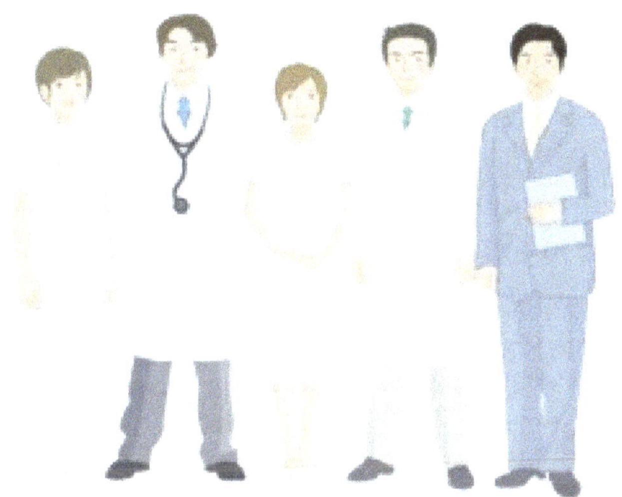

When it comes to managing Polycystic Ovary Syndrome (PCOS) and the emotional challenges associated with it, healthcare providers play a crucial role in providing support and guidance. Firstly, healthcare providers, including doctors, nurses, and mental health professionals, are trained to understand the complexities of PCOS and its impact on emotional well-being. They can offer valuable information and resources to help individuals better understand their condition and cope with its effects.

One important aspect of the healthcare provider's role is to address psychological concerns related to PCOS diagnosis and management. This includes providing a safe and non-judgmental space for individuals to express their emotions, fears, and concerns about living with PCOS. Healthcare providers can listen attentively to patients' experiences, validate their feelings, and offer empathy and support.

In addition to addressing immediate psychological concerns, healthcare providers also play a key role in providing ongoing emotional support for individuals with PCOS. This may involve monitoring mental health symptoms, such as anxiety or depression, and offering appropriate interventions or referrals to mental health professionals for further evaluation and treatment.

Furthermore, healthcare providers can offer practical strategies for managing stress, anxiety, and mood fluctuations associated with PCOS. This may include recommending stress-reduction techniques, such as mindfulness, relaxation exercises, or therapy. Healthcare providers can also provide education and guidance on lifestyle modifications, such as diet, exercise, and sleep hygiene, which can have a positive impact on mental well-being. Healthcare providers can address the emotional impact of hair-related concerns, such as hirsutism (excessive hair growth) or hair loss, on self-image and confidence. They can offer empathetic listening, validate patients' feelings, and provide information about available treatment options for managing hair-related symptoms.

By offering empathy, education, and practical strategies for coping with emotional challenges, healthcare providers can empower patients to better manage their condition and improve their overall quality of life.

CHAPTER 7:

DIY RECIPES TO MANAGE PCOS AND HAIR HEALTH

1. Recipes for Hormonal Balance in PCOS
2. Recipes for Hair Loss in PCOS
3. Recipes for Hirsutism in PCOS

The concept of using do-it-yourself (DIY) recipes for PCOS management involves harnessing the power of natural remedies and homemade treatments to address the underlying hormonal imbalances and alleviate associated symptoms. By utilizing ingredients readily available in our kitchens or local grocery stores, individuals with PCOS can take an active role in their health and well-being.

One of the key benefits of DIY recipes for PCOS management is their natural and holistic approach. Unlike conventional treatments that may come with side effects or risks, DIY recipes often utilize natural ingredients that are gentle on the body and promote overall health. Additionally, DIY recipes can be tailored to individual preferences and needs, allowing for a personalized approach to PCOS management.

RECIPES FOR HORMONAL BALANCE IN PCOS

Hormonal balance plays a crucial role in managing PCOS symptoms, and DIY recipes can be a natural and effective way to support this balance. Here are some homemade recipes aimed at promoting hormonal harmony in individuals with PCOS:

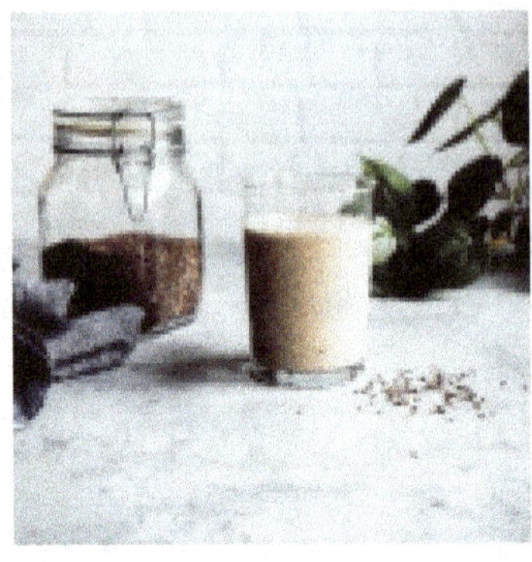

Flaxseed Smoothie:

Blend 1 tablespoon of ground flaxseeds with mixed berries, spinach, almond milk, and a scoop of protein powder.

Flaxseeds are rich in omega-3 fatty acids and lignans, which can help regulate hormone levels and improve insulin sensitivity.

Cinnamon Tea:

Steep a cinnamon stick in hot water for 10-15 minutes.

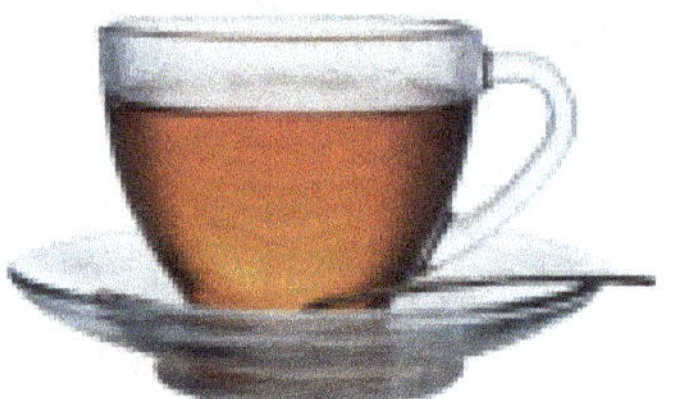

Cinnamon is known for its anti-inflammatory properties and ability to regulate blood sugar levels, which can help balance hormones in PCOS.

Spearmint Infusion:

Steep fresh spearmint leaves in boiling water for 5-10 minutes, then strain.

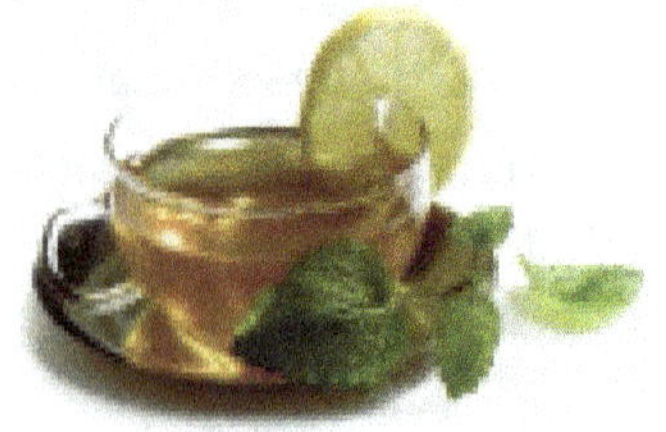

Spearmint has anti-androgenic properties and

may help reduce levels of testosterone; a hormone often elevated in PCOS.

Chia Seed Pudding:

Mix 2 tablespoons of chia seeds with coconut milk, vanilla extract, and a dash of cinnamon.

Chia seeds are high in fiber and omega-3 fatty acids, which can help regulate insulin and hormone levels.

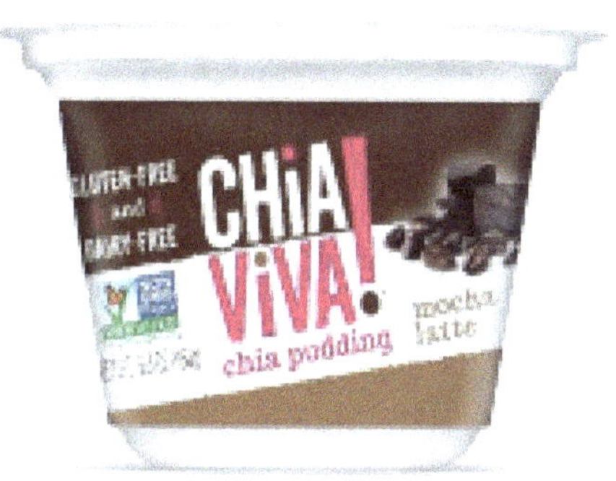

Turmeric Golden Milk:

Warm coconut milk with turmeric, ginger, cinnamon, and a pinch of black pepper.

Turmeric contains curcumin, a compound with anti-inflammatory and hormone-balancing effects.

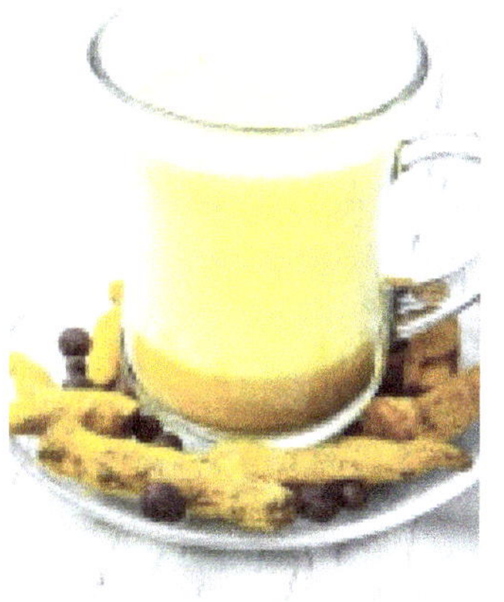

Flaxseed Crackers:

Mix ground flaxseeds with water, garlic powder, and herbs, then spread thinly on a baking sheet.

Bake until crisp to make homemade flaxseed crackers, which are rich in fiber and healthy fats.

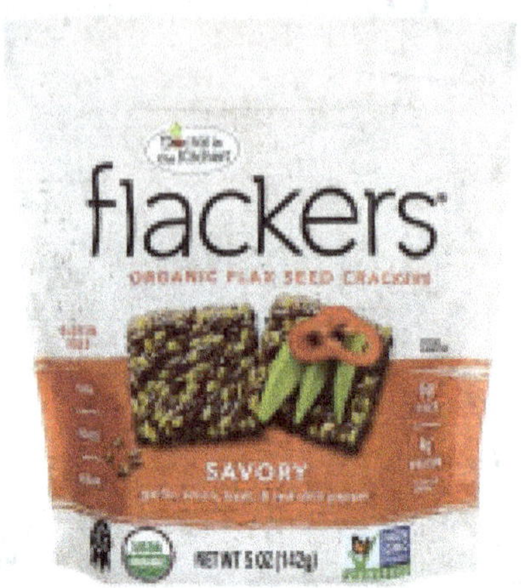

Sesame Seed Salad Dressing:

Blend sesame seeds with olive oil, lemon juice, garlic, and a touch of honey.

Sesame seeds are a good source of lignans, which may help balance hormones in PCOS.

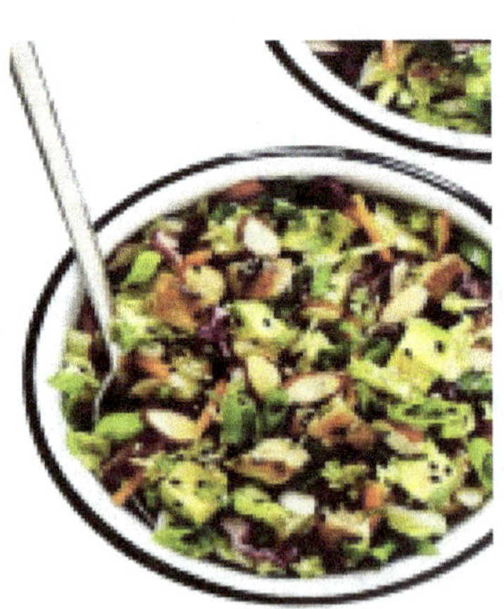

Maca Root Energy Balls:

Combine maca powder with almond butter, dates, and shredded coconut, then roll into balls.

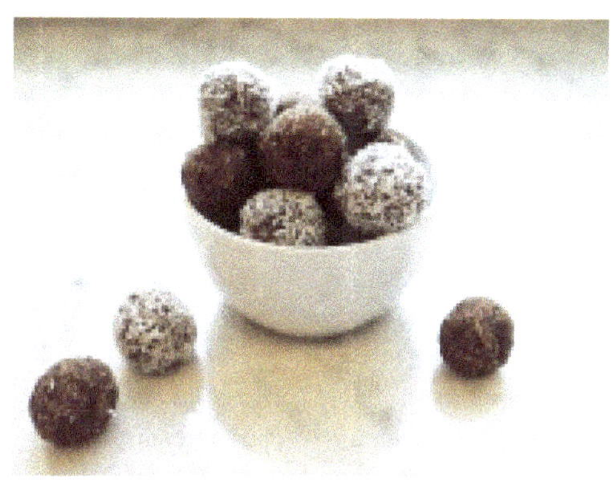

Maca root is an adaptogenic herb that may help regulate hormone levels and improve energy levels.

Hormone-Balancing Smoothie:

Blend together kale, pineapple, avocado, coconut water, and a handful of almonds.

Kale is rich in vitamins and minerals that support hormonal balance, while pineapple contains bromelain, which can help reduce inflammation.

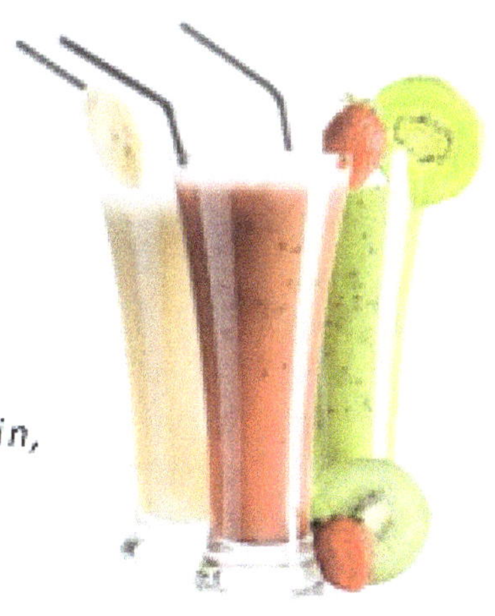

Herbal Tea Blend:

Combine equal parts of dried red clover, chasteberry (vitex), and licorice root.

Steep 1 tablespoon of the herbal blend in hot water for 10-15 minutes, then strain and enjoy. *Red clover and chasteberry are known for their hormone-balancing properties, while licorice root can support adrenal health.*

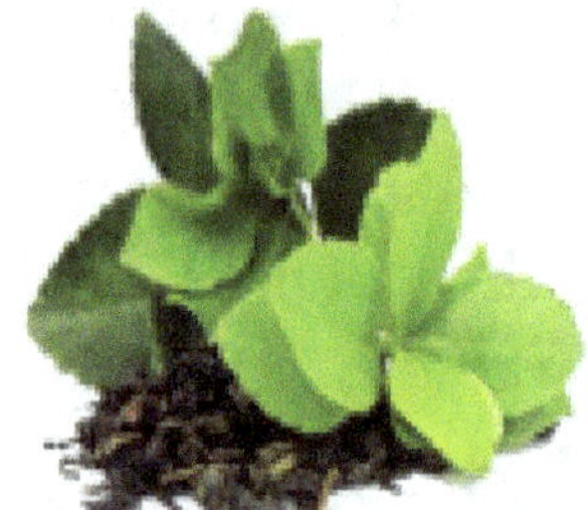

Omega-3-Rich Salad:

Toss together mixed greens, sliced cucumber, cherry tomatoes, and grilled salmon or canned sardines.

Drizzle with a dressing made from olive oil, lemon juice, and Dijon mustard.

Fatty fish like salmon and sardines are rich in omega-3 fatty acids, which can help reduce inflammation and support hormone balance.

Pumpkin Seed Trail Mix:

Combine raw pumpkin seeds with almonds, walnuts, dried cranberries, and a sprinkle of cinnamon.

Portion into individual servings for a convenient snack that provides protein, healthy fats, and hormone-balancing nutrients.

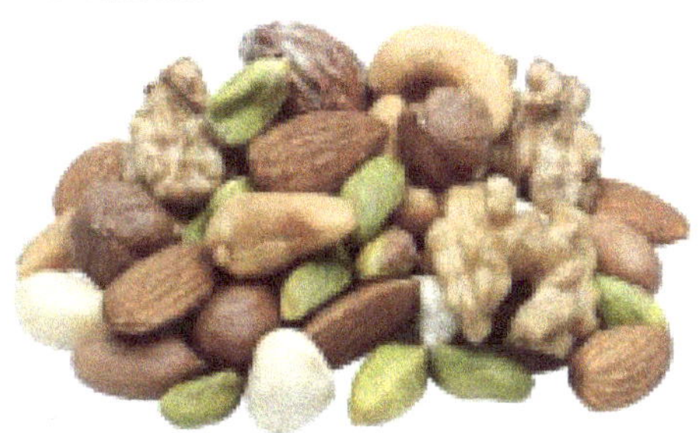

Hormone-
Balancing Soup:

Simmer onions, garlic, celery, carrots, lentils, and leafy greens in vegetable broth until tender. Season with turmeric, cumin, and paprika for added flavor and hormone-balancing benefits. *Lentils are a good source of fiber and plant-based protein, which can help stabilize blood sugar levels and support hormone balance.*

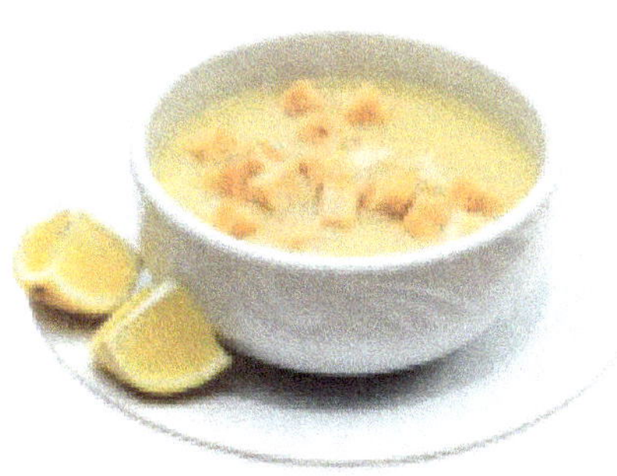

Hormone-Balancing Overnight Oats:

Combine rolled oats with chia seeds, almond milk, Greek yogurt, and a dash of cinnamon.

Refrigerate overnight and top with fresh berries and a drizzle of honey before serving.

Chia seeds are rich in fiber and omega-3 fatty acids, which can help regulate hormone levels and promote satiety.

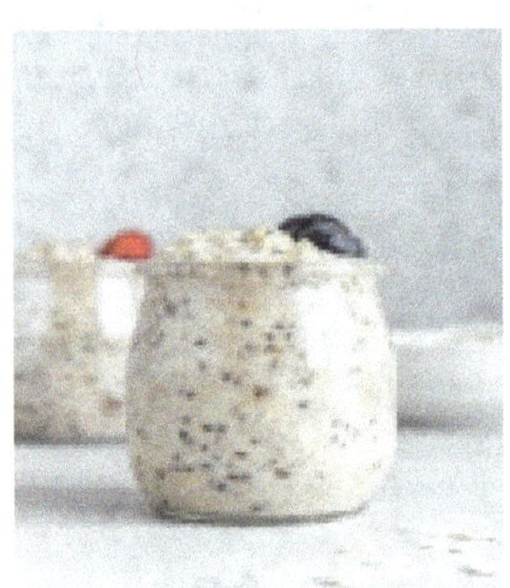

DIY RECIPES FOR HAIR LOSS

Rosemary Infused Oil:

Combine dried rosemary leaves with olive or coconut oil in a jar.

Let the mixture sit for several days to allow the oil to infuse with the rosemary scent and properties.

Massage the infused oil into the scalp regularly to stimulate hair follicles and promote growth.

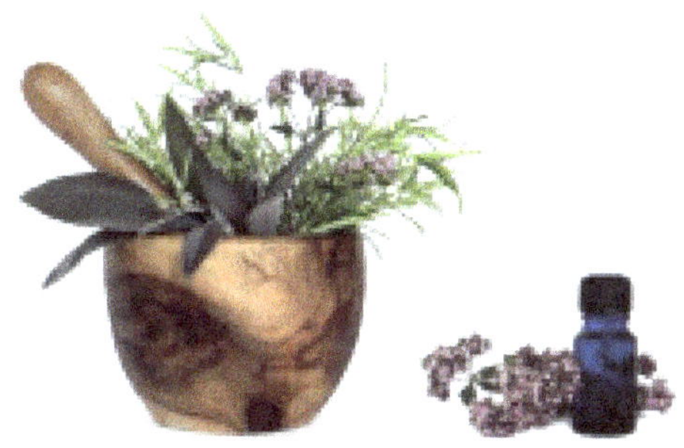

Egg Hair Mask:

Whisk together one egg with a tablespoon of olive oil until well combined.

Apply the mixture to clean, damp hair and scalp, focusing on areas of thinning or loss.

Leave the mask on for 20-30 minutes before rinsing with cool water and shampooing as usual. The protein in eggs helps strengthen hair strands and promote growth.

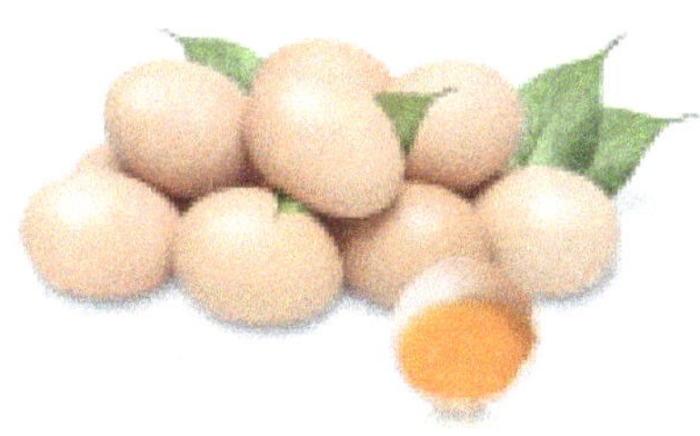

Aloe Vera Scalp Treatment:

Extract fresh aloe vera gel from an aloe leaf and massage it directly onto the scalp.

Leave the gel on for 30 minutes to an hour before rinsing with lukewarm water.

Aloe vera has soothing and hydrating properties that can help reduce inflammation and promote a healthy scalp environment for hair growth.

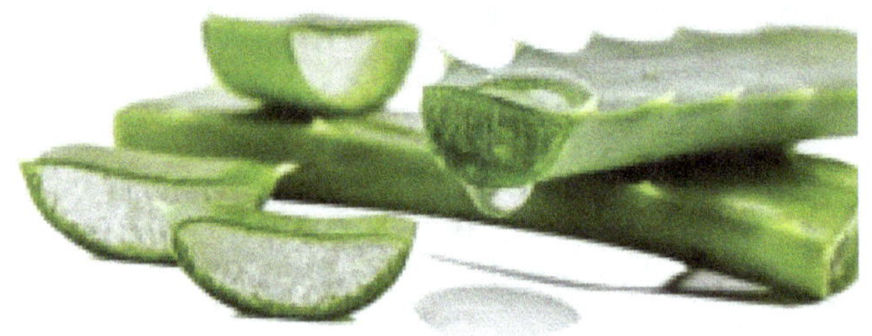

Onion Juice Hair Rinse:

Blend a fresh onion into a smooth paste, then strain the juice using a cheesecloth or fine sieve.

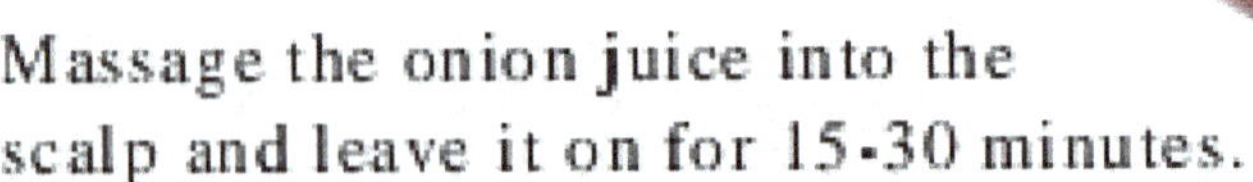

Massage the onion juice into the scalp and leave it on for 15-30 minutes.

Rinse the hair thoroughly with water to remove the onion odor. Onion juice contains sulfur, which may help stimulate hair follicles and promote growth.

Coconut Milk Hair Mask:

Mix coconut milk with a few drops of essential oil (such as lavender or rosemary) for fragrance and additional benefits.

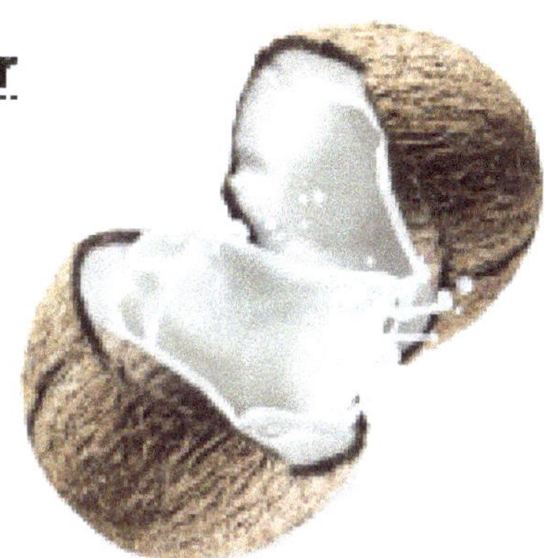

Apply the mixture to the scalp and hair, focusing on areas of thinning or loss.

Leave the mask on for 30-60 minutes before rinsing with water and shampooing as usual. Coconut milk is rich in vitamins and minerals that nourish the scalp and hair follicles.

Green Tea Hair Rinse:

Brew a strong cup of green tea and let it cool to room temperature.

Pour the green tea over clean, damp hair and massage it into the scalp.

Leave the rinse on for 10-15 minutes before rinsing with water. Green tea contains antioxidants and catechins that can help stimulate hair growth and prevent loss.

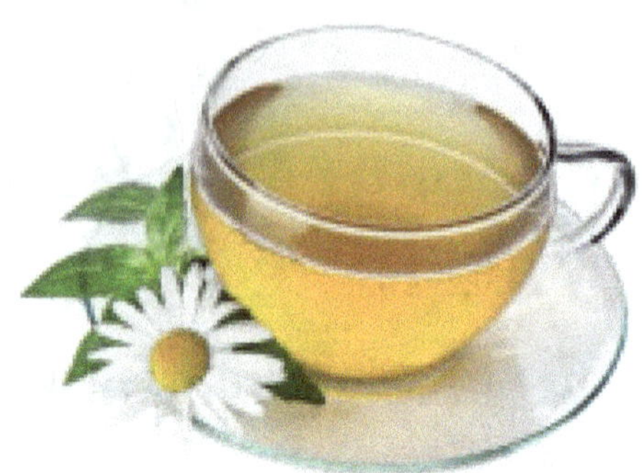

Fenugreek Seed Hair Mask:

Soak fenugreek seeds in water overnight, then blend them into a paste.

Apply the fenugreek paste to the scalp and hair, covering all areas evenly.

Leave the mask on for 30-60 minutes before rinsing with water and shampooing as usual. Fenugreek seeds are rich in proteins and nicotinic acid, which may help strengthen hair and promote growth.

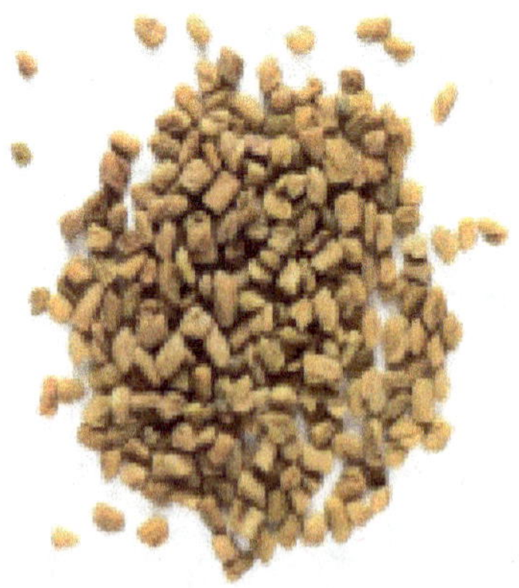

Castor Oil Scalp Massage:

Warm up castor oil slightly and massage it into the scalp using circular motions.

Leave the oil on overnight for maximum absorption, covering the hair with a shower cap or towel.

In the morning, shampoo the hair thoroughly to remove the oil. Castor oil contains ricin oleic acid, which has anti-inflammatory and antimicrobial properties that can help improve scalp health and stimulate hair growth.

Avocado Hair Mask:

Mash a ripe avocado and mix it with a tablespoon of honey and a tablespoon of olive oil.

Apply the mixture to clean, damp hair and scalp, covering all areas thoroughly.

Leave the mask on for 30-45 minutes before rinsing with lukewarm water and shampooing as usual. Avocado is rich in vitamins E and B, which can help moisturize and strengthen hair, reducing breakage and promoting growth.

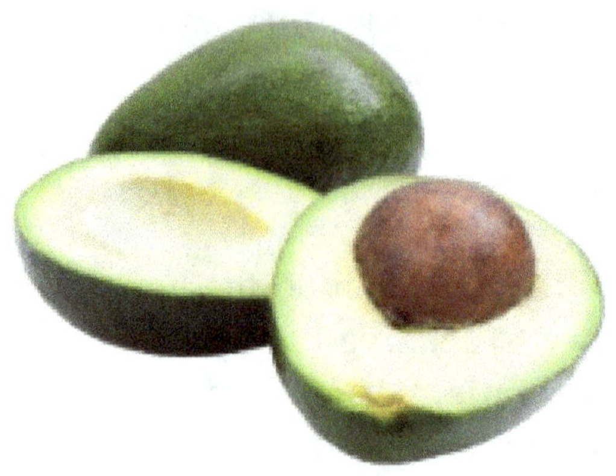

Hibiscus Hair Rinse:

Steep dried hibiscus flowers in hot water for 20-30 minutes, then strain the liquid.

Use the hibiscus infusion as a final rinse after shampooing and conditioning.

Leave the rinse on for a few minutes before rinsing with cool water. Hibiscus contains antioxidants and vitamins that can help nourish the scalp and strengthen hair follicles, promoting growth and preventing breakage.

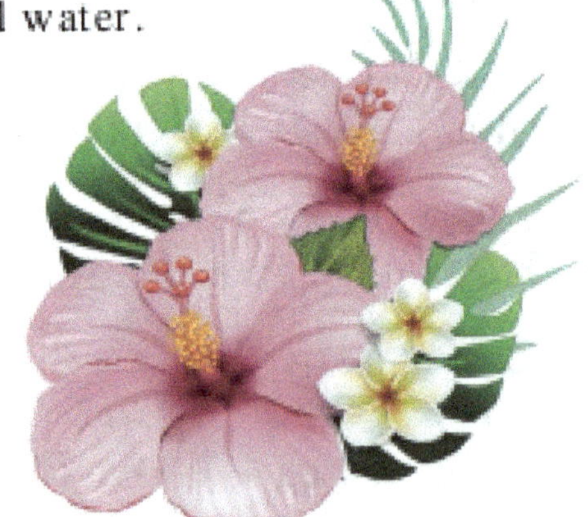

DIY RECIPES FOR HIRSUTISM

Spearmint Tea:

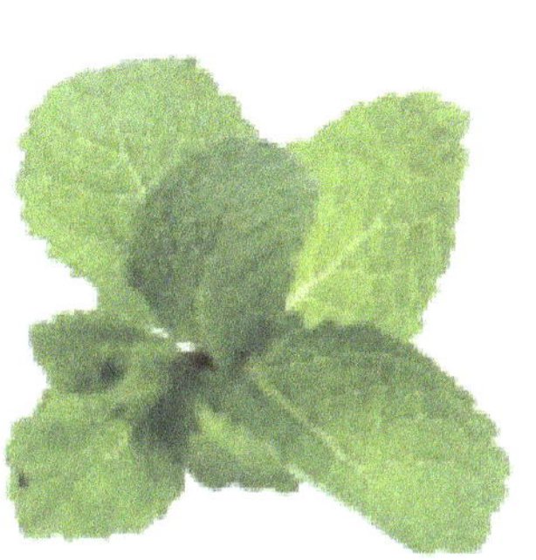

Steep fresh or dried spearmint leaves in hot water for 5-10 minutes.

Drink 1-2 cups daily to help reduce levels of testosterone, which can contribute to hirsutism.

Turmeric Face Mask:

Mix 1 tablespoon of turmeric powder with yogurt or honey to form a paste.

Apply the mask to areas of excess hair growth and leave on for 15-20 minutes before rinsing off.

Turmeric has anti-inflammatory properties that can help soothe the skin and reduce hair growth.

Sugar Waxing Paste:

Mix 2 cups of sugar, 1/4 cup of lemon juice, and 1/4 cup of water in a saucepan.

Heat the mixture over medium heat until it reaches a thick, amber-colored consistency.

Let the wax cool slightly, then apply to the skin in the direction of hair growth and quickly pull it off in the opposite direction.

Sugar waxing is a natural hair removal method that can help reduce the appearance of unwanted hair over time.

Green Tea Facial Toner:

Brew a cup of green tea and let it cool completely.

Pour the green tea into a spray bottle and store it in the refrigerator.

Spritz the toner onto clean skin twice a day to help reduce inflammation and regulate sebum production.

Oatmeal and Honey Scrub:

Mix 1/2 cup of ground oats with 2 tablespoons of honey to form a thick paste.

Gently massage the scrub onto damp skin in circular motions for 2-3 minutes, then rinse off with warm water.

Oatmeal helps exfoliate the skin and remove dead cells, while honey has antimicrobial properties that can help prevent ingrown hairs.

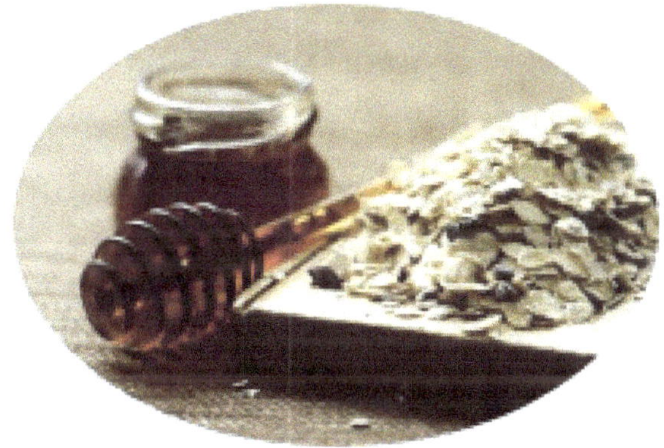

Lavender Essential Oil Blend:

Dilute 5-10 drops of lavender essential oil in 1 tablespoon of carrier oil, such as coconut or almond oil.

Apply the oil blend to areas of excess hair growth and massage it into the skin twice daily.

Lavender oil has calming properties that can help reduce stress, which may contribute to hormonal imbalances associated with hirsutism.

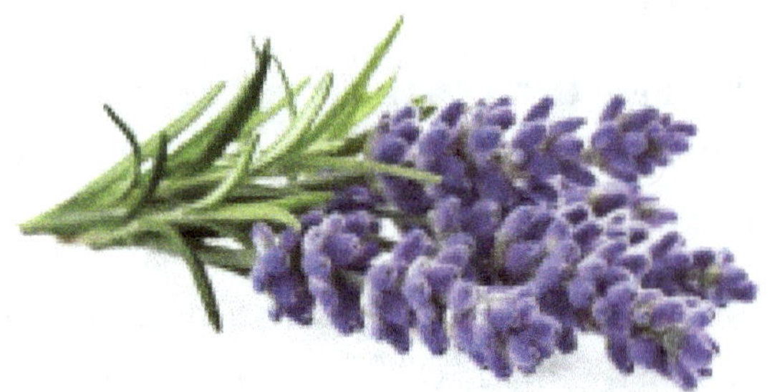

Chamomile Hair Removal Paste:

Mix equal parts of chamomile tea and chickpea flour to form a thick paste.

Apply the paste to the skin in the direction of hair growth and leave it on for 15-20 minutes before rinsing off with warm water.

Chamomile has anti-inflammatory properties that can help soothe the skin and reduce redness associated with hair removal.

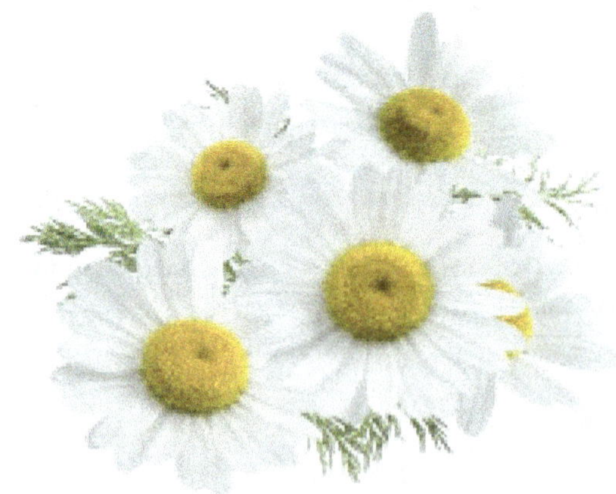

Papaya Hair Mask:

Mash ripe papaya into a smooth paste and apply it to areas of excess hair growth.

Leave the mask on for 15-20 minutes before rinsing off with lukewarm water.

Papaya contains an enzyme called papain, which can help weaken hair follicles and reduce hair growth over time.

Apple Cider Vinegar Rinse:

Mix equal parts of apple cider vinegar and water in a spray bottle.

Spritz the mixture onto clean skin and let it air dry.

Apple cider vinegar helps balance the skin's pH levels and can help prevent ingrown hairs.

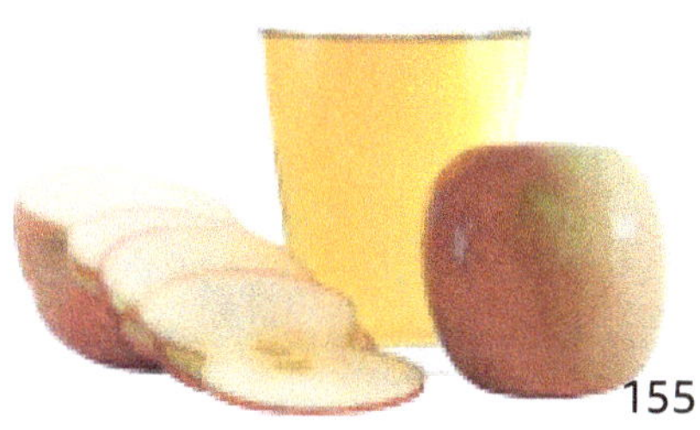

Rosewater and Witch Hazel Toner:

Mix equal parts of rosewater and witch hazel in a spray bottle.

Spritz the toner onto clean skin twice a day to help tighten pores and reduce inflammation.

Witch hazel has astringent properties that can help soothe irritated skin and reduce redness.

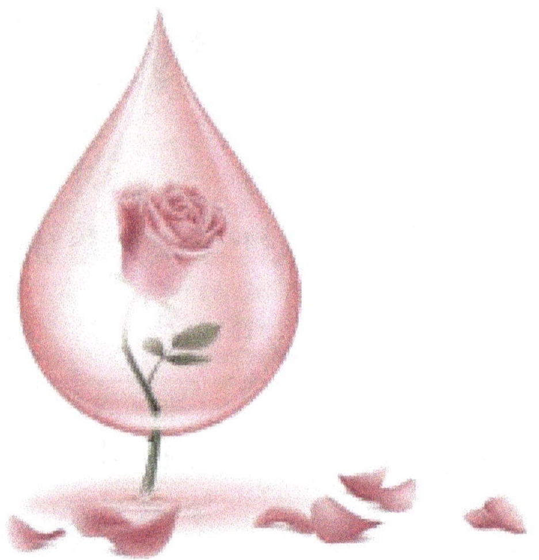

<u>CONCLUSION</u>

In conclusion, "PCOS and Hair Harmony" aims to empower individuals with polycystic ovary syndrome (PCOS) to take control of their hair health and overall well-being. Throughout this book, we've explored the complex relationship between PCOS and hair issues, from hair loss to hirsutism, and provided practical strategies and DIY recipes for managing these symptoms naturally.

We've delved into the underlying hormonal imbalances that contribute to hair-related concerns in PCOS and offered insights into how lifestyle changes, dietary adjustments, and holistic approaches can help restore hormonal balance and promote healthy hair growth.

By understanding the root causes of hair issues in PCOS and implementing targeted interventions, readers can embark on a journey towards reclaiming confidence and embracing their unique beauty. Remember, managing PCOS and achieving hair harmony is not a one-size-fits-all approach, but rather a personalized journey guided by self-awareness, patience, and resilience.

As we conclude this book, let us remember that the path to hair harmony is not without its challenges, but with knowledge, support, and determination, it is indeed attainable. May this book serve as a beacon of hope and empowerment for all those navigating the complexities of PCOS and seeking harmony in their hair and their lives.

USEFULL WEBSITES

There's a lot of information on the internet, but it's important to be cautious. Many medical websites focus on the most severe cases of disorders. For example, with PCOS, most women have mild or moderate symptoms, while only a few have severe symptoms. Some may not even have any symptoms at all. Only a small percentage of women with PCOS experience very irregular periods. It's important to remember that people with severe problems are more likely to be active in online chat rooms, so their experiences might not represent everyone's. Look for websites from reputable sources like universities, government bodies, or large hospitals. I couldn't find one website that covers everything about PCOS, but there are some good sites that focus on different aspects of it. Here are a few of my favorites that you might find helpful too.

- **American Congress of Obstetricians and Gynecologists (ACOG):** https://www.acog.org/womens-health/faqs/polycystic-ovary-syndrome-pcos

- **National Institutes of Health (NIH):** https://www.nichd.nih.gov/health/topics/pcos/Pages/default.aspx

- **Mayo Clinic:** https://www.mayoclinic.org/

- **National Health Service (NHS), UK:** https://www.nhs.uk/conditions/polycystic-ovary-syndrome-pcos/

- **The Polycystic Ovary Syndrome Association (PCOSAA):** https://www.pcosaa.org/

- **PCOS Living:** https://www.pcosliving.com/

- **The National PCOS Association:** https://pcoschallenge.org/

- **American Academy of Dermatology (AAD):** https://www.aad.org/public